How to Survive Outpatient Hemodialysis:

A Guide for Patients with Kidney Failure

Steven L. Belcher
RN, MSN, MS

Published by Walters Publishing from
BLUE ARTISTS, LLC

Copyright © 2020 Steven L. Belcher
All rights reserved.
Published by Walters Publishing from
BLUE ARTISTS, LLC

Printed in the United States of America.

This publication may not be reproduced, stored in a retrieval system, or transmitted in whole or in part, in any form or by any means, electronic, mechanical, photocopying, recording, or otherwise, without the prior written permission of Steven L. Belcher or Walters Publishing from Blue Artists, LLC, the representing agency. To order additional copies of *How to Survive Outpatient Hemodialysis*, please visit urbankidneyalliance.org

This publication is designed to provide accurate and authoritative information in regard to the subject matter covered. It is sold with the understanding that the publisher is not engaged in rendering legal, accounting, or another professional service. If legal advice or other expert assistance is required, the services of a competent professional person should be sought.

Contents

Preface 7

Introduction 9

Chapter 1 What Is Chronic Kidney Failure? 13

Chapter 2 Introduction to Hemodialysis 17

Chapter 3 Your First Day at Outpatient Hemodialysis 33

Chapter 4 Patients Rights and Responsibilities 41

Chapter 5 Understanding Patient Grievance Policy 45

Chapter 6 Treatment Options for Kidney Failure: Hemodialysis and Peritoneal Dialysis 49

Chapter 7 Treatment Options for Kidney Failure: Kidney Transplants 61

Chapter 8 How to Care for Your Access 75

Chapter 9 Making Wise Food Choices 85

Chapter 10 Additional Important Information 95

Chapter 11 Stay Healthy 115

Chapter 12 Coronavirus and Kidney Disease 119

Acknowledgments 127

Glossary 135

Online Resources for Patients 151

Foreword
By Ken Sutha and Charles A. Bonner

Ken Sutha

I first learned about Steve Belcher and his advocacy for kidney patients through the series of educational livestreams he produces and hosts for Urban Kidney Alliance. For those not familiar, Urban Kidney Alliance is a grassroots non-profit group whose mission is to educate and increase awareness about kidney disease, particularly in urban communities. I was invited as a guest for one of their shows to share my experiences as a patient, having myself lived through kidney disease, dialysis, and transplantation, and now also as a pediatric nephrologist taking care of patients going through these same things. The patient-partnered education that the Urban Kidney Alliance and Steve does is vitally important, and it is critical in addressing the hidden epidemic of kidney disease, particularly within minority communities that are at even greater risk for facing kidney disease. According to the National Kidney Foundation, one in three American adults is at risk for developing kidney disease, but still the majority of those with kidney disease don't even know it. As a pediatrician and a nephrologist, I am well aware of how social determinants of health, disparities in access to healthcare, and systemic racism have resulted in increased risk of chronic kidney disease, later diagnosis, and ultimately the need for dialysis in patients from urban communities and for Black and Latino patients in particular. As a kidney patient, I am also all too familiar with how overwhelming a new diagnosis of kidney disease or the transition to dialysis can be.

In creating this guide for new dialysis patients, Steve builds upon the fantastic advocacy and educational resources he has compiled in his work with the Urban Kidney Alliance. Even as a seasoned kidney patient of over two decades and a kidney doctor myself, the process of walking into the dialysis clinic for the first time, meeting an entirely new care team, and learning the ins and outs of dialysis treatment was intimidating and a lot for me to take in, reminding me a bit of the first day of school. As I settled in and got to know my dialysis team, I definitely got more comfortable, but without a doubt, I would have loved to have a resource like this guide to give me a heads up about the unknowns of dialysis—including what to expect in this new environment and ideas about what kinds of questions I should ask about my treatment. Though this guide is targeted at new outpatient hemodialysis patients, it contains valuable information for all patients facing kidney failure. Steve's firsthand experience and expertise from years as a dialysis nurse provides so many insights about the details of the day to day running of dialysis that many nephrologists may not even know. With this guide and Steve's expertise in your pocket, you will be well prepared to approach the unknowns of dialysis for the first time, including highlights of the basics of kidney failure, who you will expect to meet as part of your dialysis team, other options available for kidney replacement treatment, and special considerations for kidney and dialysis patients during the COVID-19 pandemic.

Ken Sutha, MD, PhD
Pediatric Nephrologist
Kidney Patient for 28 Years

***

Charles A. Bonner

I recently met Steve Belcher on a Zoom meeting call about kidney failure and dialysis. To be specific, it was one of Steve's live broadcast shows, where he encourages his viewers to be informed about the ins and outs of their dialysis treatment and to advocate for themselves. Most importantly, his shows raise awareness about preventing and screening for kidney disease.

This would prove to be a fortunate encounter, as two to three days prior I received news that one of my best friends and high school classmates was in the hospital with kidney failure. "For certain, he would need dialysis and maybe a kidney transplant," a mutual friend and classmate informed me. After expressing my surprise and shock, I felt helpless that I could not offer any suggestions, recommendations, or help to my sick classmate at the time.

Luckily, after interacting with Steve during the Zoom meeting, he followed up with me and emailed me his manuscript, *How to Survive Outpatient Hemodialysis: A Guide For Patients with Kidney Failure*. I devoured Steve's book. "Wow!" I exclaimed as I read it. He calls this a "guide," but this is more like the Bible for anyone grappling with kidney failure and seeking to maintain sanity with all the unknowns of starting dialysis.

My experience with Steve's book was like having a medical expert in my social circle. Steve's excellent bedside manner and anticipatory guidance shines through in *How to Survive Outpatient Hemodialysis* as it reflects the depth, nature, and extent of his knowledge practicing as a RN in the dialysis field for thirty-three years. Written in a plain and concise manner, Steve's "guide" details all the information I could wish to share with my classmate, terrified about his diagnosis and eager to understand what to expect if he decided to undergo dialysis.

I've been a trial lawyer for forty years, and juries, like patients, need complex information distilled into simple, understandable narratives, grabbing the attention of their evolutionary brains that are pre-wired for story. With my commitments in the areas of civil rights and human rights, it was easy for me to connect with Steve's drive in *How to Survive Outpatient Dialysis*. Readers will easily connect with Steve's drive as well. This book will serve as a means for all kidney failure patients to be informed as a patient, so they can advocate for themselves and make the best healthcare decisions in collaboration with their medical team.

Charles A. Bonner, Esq.
Attorney at Law
Author of *The Bracelet: The Story to End Child Sex Slavery in the World* and *The Tip of the Arrow: The Selma Student Nonviolent Civil Rights Movement, A Study in Leadership*

Preface

I was inspired to write *How to Survive Outpatient Hemodialysis: A Guide for Patients with Kidney Failure* for, mainly, three focal reasons. The first reason is that more than 750,000 patients per year in the United States are affected by kidney failure. In fact, nine out of ten adults have chronic kidney failure and don't even know they have it. By the time they find out, it's often too late to do anything about it, making dialysis inevitable. This scenario gives a person little to no time to adjust to this new and life-changing event. The second reason is to assure that patients who are diagnosed with kidney failure and beginning outpatient hemodialysis for the first time will have the information necessary to adjust to outpatient hemodialysis. Third, it is my hope that such a guide will help patients effectively navigate the admission process on the first day of arrival for outpatient dialysis treatment. Many patients walk through the doors of the dialysis clinic for the first time with no idea of what to expect from the process, let alone on their first day of treatment. Patients receive so much information on the first day of dialysis that most tend to forget what they're told. That's why the first day of dialysis can be so overwhelming for patients—the unknown leaves them in the dark, not knowing what to expect. Some patients experience a wide range of emotions, such as anxiety, depression, apprehension, and a general sense of being unwell because of the disease. Let this book serve as an approachable reference guide for kidney patients and their family members attending outpatient hemodialysis.

Introduction

So the day has finally arrived for you to attend outpatient hemodialysis for the first time at one of the thousands of dialysis clinics across the United States. Know that you are not alone in this journey. Kidney failure affects almost 750,000 people per year in the United States. During my ten years as a dialysis technician and twenty-three years as a charge nurse, I've admitted many new patients for outpatient dialysis who were overwhelmed—either by the admission intake process or by the heaps of information given to them on the first day about the dialysis process, or both. If patients and their family or caregivers miss out on vital information they may need to refer to in the future, information that will help them manage their dialysis treatment, this overwhelm can become a serious problem.

I wrote this guide to help eliminate or lessen any fears experienced by patients starting outpatient dialysis treatment for the first time, and to give you the information needed to remain healthy on hemodialysis. Another purpose for writing this guide is to provide you with information and knowledge on ways to manage what's going on with your dialysis treatment. This book focuses on incenter hemodialysis, but it has useful information for peritoneal dialysis and home hemodialysis patients as well. As of my writing this, I could not find any books that provide an overview of what to expect from the outpatient dialysis center as a new patient. This guide explains what you need to know and what takes place when starting outpatient hemodialysis. Some details in this guide may vary from clinic to clinic, doctor to doctor, but information in this guide will apply to most people. I recommend that you talk with your dialysis team and ask any questions and have them explain to you any difference from what's discussed in this guide that you may see or experience in your clinic.

New patients who begin outpatient hemodialysis for the first time are usually not prepared for the busy-ness of the hemodialysis unit. They are often taken aback when entering the treatment area for the first time. Some patients compare their first time in a dialysis treatment area during patient shift change as being in a "factory plant." In addition, units usually do not give dialysis staff the time to sit with patients during treatment to educate them about their treatment.

Introduction

After you start outpatient hemodialysis and decide that this option is not for you, there is the option of home hemodialysis, which is offered by most dialysis companies. I discuss more on home hemodialysis in chapter 6. This book is divided into ten chapters packed with insightful, robust information to help you adjust and adapt to your new reality.

Chapter 1 begins with a definition of chronic kidney failure and the different treatment options for chronic kidney failure. **Chapter 2** introduces you to hemodialysis and what to expect from it. **Chapter 3** takes you into the outpatient clinic and shows you what to expect on your first day. **Chapter 4** helps you understand your rights and responsibilities as an end-stage kidney disease patient. **Chapter 5** explores the patient grievance policy and what you need to know if you have an issue with your treatment center. **Chapter 6** explores and explains two treatment options for kidney failure in detail: hemodialysis and peritoneal dialysis. **Chapter 7** explores and explains another treatment option for kidney failure in detail: transplantation. **Chapter 8** talks about how to care for your dialysis access and what else you need to know about your access. **Chapter 9** discusses making wise food choices to help you live a healthy life on hemodialysis. **Chapter 10** gives you other need-to-know information about dialysis. **Chapter 11** provides information on how to maintain a healthy lifestyle while undergoing hemodialysis. **Chapter 12** talks about what you need to know regarding coronavirus and kidney disease.

Many of you may not be prepared to read this book from cover to cover. That is perfectly fine. You can go straight to any chapter that interests you and learn what you are most interested in from that chapter. Some of the topics I will discuss may be unfamiliar to you, but don't let that keep you from learning all you can about your dialysis treatment and care. In addition, I've included an alphabetical kidney failure glossary, which defines words that are often used when healthcare team members talk or write about kidney failure and its treatment. It is designed for people whose kidneys have failed and for their families and friends. The knowledge and information you get from this book will not only help you understand how to care for yourself having kidney disease but also help you get the most of your hemodialysis treatment and maintain a healthy lifestyle while undergoing outpatient hemodialysis.

Chapter 1

What Is Chronic Kidney Failure?

In order to understand what chronic kidney failure is, you have to know some basic functions of your kidneys—also known as the renal system—and how changes in the normal function lead to kidney failure.

We each have two kidneys, and they serve as very important organs. There is one kidney located on each side of the backbone, each extending a little below the ribs. They weigh four to six ounces and are a little bigger than your fist. Kidneys are responsible for maintaining a delicate balance of water and certain chemicals known as electrolytes in your body. Without this balance, your other organs cannot function properly. The kidneys also act as a chemical system to remove waste and maintain a healthy chemical balance in your blood.

Major Functions of the Normal Kidneys

1. Remove waste from the blood

2. Remove excess water from the body
3. Regulate blood pressure
4. Control red blood cell production
5. Regulate bone health

What Is Chronic Kidney Failure?

Chronic kidney failure is a result of the most serious kidney diseases. And if you're undergoing chronic kidney failure, you may have felt fine for the past few years, but chances are you've had kidney problems for a much longer period of time. That's because it's a slow, long process, one that involves a continual loss of nephrons, the working units of the kidney. In each kidney, there are over two million nephrons. At least 75% of them must be damaged to cause obvious illness.

It can take many years to go from chronic kidney failure to end-stage renal disease (ESRD). Urine formation begins in a part of the nephron called the glomerulus, a group of very fine blood vessels. When the heart pumps blood, it builds up pressure in these vessels. The pressure forces about 200 quarts of fluid from the blood through the glomerulus into a small tube. All this fluid is not lost; most is reabsorbed. What is lost is called urine, which is the excess water and chemicals that the body doesn't need.

Chapter 1: What Is Chronic Kidney Failure?

Treatment Options for Kidney Failure

You have three options for treating kidney disease:

1. Hemodialysis
2. Peritoneal Dialysis
3. Kidney Transplant

    a) Living related donor

    6) Living unrelated donor

    b) Deceased donor kidney

Which option is best for you? That choice depends on many different factors. Hopefully, up to this point, you have been involved in making the decision that led you to select hemodialysis. Some patients may change from one mode of dialysis to another as their needs change. I encourage you to talk with your kidney doctor about the options available to you.

Below is a brief review of terms related to treatment options. See chapter 6 and chapter 7 for more detailed information.

Dialysis

The term used when referring to the treatment necessary for people with kidney failure. Normally, water and waste products are removed from the body by the kidneys in the form of urine. When the kidneys have stopped functioning, they cannot get rid of waste products, so dialysis treatment replaces some of the kidney's function. There are two forms of dialysis: hemodialysis and peritoneal dialysis.

Hemodialysis

A procedure that removes water and waste products from the blood by way of a catheter in a major blood vessel, or the creation of a fistula under your skin (usually in an arm) called an access. The blood is carried from your access and filtered through an artificial kidney then returned to the body cleaned.

Peritoneal Dialysis

A procedure that removes excess water and waste products via the abdomen. Instead of using an artificial kidney to do the filtering, this procedure uses the person's own membranes found in the abdominal area for filtering purposes. CAPD, another form of peritoneal dialysis, refers to a continuous peritoneal dialysis procedure.

Kidney Transplantation

The third option for patients with kidney failure. Transplants are performed by surgically removing a functioning kidney from a relative, a friend, an altruistic donor, or someone who recently died and implanting it into the person with kidney failure.

Chapter 2

Introduction to Hemodialysis

What Is Hemodialysis?

Hemodialysis cleans and filters your blood using a machine to temporarily rid your body of harmful wastes, extra salt, and extra water. Hemodialysis helps control blood pressure and helps your body keep the proper balance of important electrolytes, such as potassium, sodium, calcium, and bicarbonate.

How Does It Work?

Hemodialysis uses a special filter called a dialyzer that functions as an artificial kidney to clean your blood. During treatment, your blood travels through tubes into the dialyzer, which filters out wastes and extra water. The cleaned blood flows through another set of tubes back into your body. The dialyzer is connected to a machine that monitors blood flow and removes waste from the blood.

Hemodialysis is usually needed three times a week, and each treatment lasts from three to five hours—

sometimes longer. During treatment you can read, write, sleep, talk, or watch television.

The Renal Team

There are many people needed to run a dialysis unit. The primary group of people involved in your care at outpatient dialysis is called a renal team. You should be introduced to them during your next several treatments. They are there to assist you with all your hemodialysis-related needs. The renal team consists of the following team members:

Nephrologist

A kidney doctor who sees you at the clinic. The nephrologist and nurse practitioner (see below) take care of problems related to your kidney disease and work closely to see that you get the greatest benefit from your dialysis. The nephrologist orders your dialysis treatments. This entails selecting the length and weekly frequency of your dialysis sessions, as well as the targeted amount of fluid to be removed (dry weight) and the dialysis concentrate that is necessary to "clean" the blood.

Nurse Practitioner

A registered nurse who returns to college for extra training in caring for people with chronic conditions, such as patients with kidney disease. They have a master's degree in nursing and are certified to write prescriptions and order diagnostic tests. In some dialysis units, the nurse practitioners treat patients in partnership with the nephrologist (kidney doctor) and provide care that has to do with your dialysis needs. This includes treating high blood pressure, anemia (low red blood cell count), and bone disease related to kidney failure.

Charge Nurse

The charge nurse coordinates the activities of the dialysis unit, assigns work to the nursing staff, and institutes emergency procedures as necessary. The charge nurse also communicates patient status to the kidney doctor as necessary.

Nursing Staff

The nursing staff is made up of registered nurses and dialysis technicians. These team members have special training in dialysis and the care of patients with kidney disease. You may have different dialysis nurses and technicians caring for you at each treatment. However, you should have one nurse, called your primary nurse, assigned to you. The primary nurse develops patient nursing care plans and sees that the patient's learning needs are met.

Social Worker

The social worker's primary role is to help you in your overall adjustment to dialysis. Like the nurse practitioner, they have a master's degree, and they should complete an initial psychosocial assessment with you to learn your individual needs, which should include your insurance, financial resources, transportation needs, living situation, and social support, as well as education and employment history and/or goals. The social worker should be available to provide education, counseling, and resource referral services as needed, and should help you arrange hemodialysis when you travel or go on vacation. They usually need at least two to three weeks' notice to make arrangements.

Dietician

The renal dietitian works closely with your kidney doctor, social worker, and charge nurse and may make recommendations for changes in some of your medications as well as diet. They have either a bachelor's or master's degree in nutrition and dietetics, are registered with the American Dietetic Association, and have extensive training in therapeutic diets for the treatment of diseases. The dietician should be available to you and your nurse on the unit during your shift and/or by appointment. During your initial nutritional assessment, the dietitian will discuss your diet and weight history to determine your current nutritional state. They should then educate you and your nurse on dietary changes needed while you are on dialysis. These changes will help you plan meals that are just right for your age, gender, and disease. The dietitian should also provide you with a monthly report of your nutrition-related blood work results.

What Is a Hemodialysis Machine?

During dialysis, your blood is cleaned using a fluid called dialysate, or "bath." Waste and fluid from your blood enter the bath and are drained away. The dialysis machine controls the flow of the blood and the bath. The dialysis machine has two separate systems: the extracorporeal (outside the body) circuit and the dialysate- delivery system. The extracorporeal circuit is the tubing, blood pump, heparin (blood thinner) pump, artificial kidney, and monitors for blood flow, blood pressure, and air detection. The dialysate delivery system of the machine mixes the bath with purified water and checks to be sure it is safe to be used for dialysis.

When I worked in dialysis as a charge nurse, many patients would ask me how much blood is outside their body during dialysis treatment. I would tell them that depending on the machine and dialyzer, no more than two cups (one pint) of blood is outside their body during dialysis.

One important feature on the dialysis machine is the air detector. Air in your bloodstream is a medical emergency, so the air detector monitors and assures that air does not get into your bloodstream. The air detector is supposed to be set by the operator before each treatment. Another important feature on the dialysis machine is the blood pump. This is where staff set your blood flow rate. You may be thinking to yourself, what is a "blood pump," or flow rate? The blood flow rate (BFR) is how fast the blood pump moves your blood through the tubing. One important point about your blood flow rate is making sure your blood flow rate speed is set to the ordered speed each time you attend your dialysis treatment. The dialysate concentrate or "bath" is what the kidney doctor prescribes for your dialysis treatment. It must have the right chemicals, or it will not clean your blood well enough. Sometimes the wrong ingredients can even hurt you, so learn what concentrate your doctor has prescribed for you and check it at each dialysis treatment. The most common machine used in many clinics are the dialysis machines made by dialysis giant Fresenius

Medical Care. However, there are many other different dialysis machines used as well.

Medical Complications During Hemodialysis

During hemodialysis treatment, some (but not all) patients may experience medical complications. While undergoing hemodialysis, **vascular access** problems are the most common reason for hospitalization. Other common problems that a patient might encounter during hemodialysis include infection, blockage from clotting, and poor blood flow. These problems can keep your access from working. You may need to undergo repeated surgeries in order to get a properly functioning access. Additionally, a patient may experience side effects from hemodialysis treatments that are a result of rapid changes in your body's water and electrolyte balance during treatment. **Muscle cramps** and **hypotension** or a sudden drop in blood pressure are two common side effects. Low blood or hypotension can make you feel weak, dizzy, or sick to your stomach.

Hypotension (Low Blood Pressure)

If your blood pressure drops during dialysis, you may experience any or all of the following symptoms:

- A sudden anxious, nervous feeling

- Nausea and/or vomiting
- Dizziness or faintness
- Yawning
- Sweating
- Feeling hot
- Ringing in your ears

If you experience any of the above symptoms during your dialysis treatment, inform your nurse or technician immediately. Below are some reasons why your blood pressure may drop:

1. If your blood pressure falls after you have been on dialysis a while, it is probably due to the removal of too much fluid from your body. This is more likely to happen if you have a large amount of fluid to remove.

2. Accidental blood loss will cause low blood pressure. Blood loss may occur if your bloodlines (tubing) come apart during dialysis, or if a needle falls out. If this happens, immediately apply pressure to the site or clamp your line and alert your nurse or technician.

3. Most patients need to take their blood pressure medicines on dialysis days. If low blood pressure occurs during treatment, this can be a problem.

You may be told to adjust how you take your blood pressure medications on dialysis days if this happens. Talk with your kidney doctor if you are not sure how to approach this situation.

Treatment of Hypotension

Below is the standard treatment for hypotension, just so you're aware of it. If your blood pressure drops during dialysis, the following measures should be taken:

1. You should be placed in a lying down position with your head lower than your feet. This is called the Trendelenburg or "T-Berg" position. It promotes blood flow to your vital organs and helps to maintain a "normal" blood pressure.

2. Your nurse may decide to increase the sodium (salt) content of the dialysate fluid on the machine. Eating salty foods tends to increase blood pressure; by measuring the salt content of the dialysate fluid, the same effect can be achieved. However, this may make you more thirsty than usual, so remember to be more careful with your fluid intake.

3. The nurse or technician may choose to use an option on the dialysis machine called "minimum UFR" (minimum ultrafiltration rate). This de-

creases the "pull" that the machine exerts to draw off fluid from the body. Thus, you may not reach your **dry weight** if the nurse has to put you in minimum UFR due to low blood pressure.

4. If your blood pressure becomes very low, the nurse or technician should give you extra fluid to help increase your blood pressure. If your pressure drops during dialysis, "normal saline" should be given through your dialysis lines. If you experience low blood pressure after dialysis, you may be given chicken bouillon (because of its high sodium content) or cold water to drink. This will help raise your blood pressure. You should remain seated in your chair until the nurse or technician informs you that your blood pressure has risen to a level where it will be safe for you to leave the dialysis unit.

Fever and/or Chills

A complication that could occur during dialysis is fever and/or chills. The normal body temperature of a person is 98.6 degrees Fahrenheit. If your temperature is greater than 100 degrees Fahrenheit prior to dialysis, you may have some type of infection. The nurse should ask you to describe any symptoms you have that may indicate an infection. It is normal for your temperature to rise slightly during dialysis, but a high temperature with or without chills during dialysis may also be due to contamination in the system. If this happens, your dialysis treatment should be terminated, and **blood cultures**—blood samples that get sent to a lab to determine if there are any bacteria present that may be causing your fever—should be taken from your dialysis lines. Most likely, you'll receive antibiotics through the dialysis lines. Your dialysis access may also be cultured, particularly if you have a hemodialysis catheter. If you experience any fever and/or chills before, during, or after dialysis, inform your nurse or technician immediately.

Skin and Hair Problems

Many people on dialysis experience changes to their skin. The skin may seem more fragile, or it may bruise or even tear easily. Easy bruising occurs if your blood thinner (heparin) is too high, or if your platelet count is too low. (Another result of low platelet levels is that your gums may bleed.) Additionally, some drugs, like prednisone, cortisone, or coumadin, can increase bruising.

Dry, itching, or cracking skin is common, too. Itching can be caused by high blood levels of phosphorus. In your body, extra phosphorus can bind with calcium to form sharp itchy crystals. Other causes of itching include not enough dialysis or dry skin caused by long, hot baths that strip the skin of oils or alcohol-based products. If you only itch on dialysis, an allergy may be the cause. One type of **heparin** might make you itchy, while another does not. Bleach used to clean the dialysis chair after each treatment may also be to blame.

Some patients with kidney failure also experience hair loss. Hair is made of protein, so if you are malnourished, a few months later your hair may break more easily and fall out. In addition, hair loss can also be caused by zinc deficiency, thyroid problems, or drug reactions. It has been said that some patients have had hair loss when the dialysis clinic changes the type of **dialyzer** (artificial kidney) they use.

It's normal to feel self-conscious about any of these skin and hair problems. The good news is that many of these problems can be helped. For the skin, taking phosphate binder medication with food can help with itchiness—so can covering your chair with a blanket, if a dialysis chair cleaned with bleach is to blame. Eating high-quality protein will help with hair loss, but it takes a couple of months to see a change. You can ask your clinic dietitian about good protein sources and your doctor for other solutions.

Chapter 2: Introduction to Hemodialysis

Getting Enough Dialysis

Healthy kidneys work twenty-four hours a day, seven days a week. When kidneys stop working, dialysis does some of this work. **Adequate dialysis** is a term used to mean enough dialysis treatment to help you live long and well. Dialysis is measured in a dose, like a dose of medicine. Your kidney doctor prescribes a dose of dialysis that should keep you feeling well. The artificial kidney or dialyzer performs some of the functions of a normal kidney. To see how well you are doing on dialysis, your blood will be drawn every month to measure your labs; specifically, urea reduction ratio (URR) and Kt/V, as well as other important tests.

Dialysis removes many wastes. One product, called urea or blood urea nitrogen (BUN), is easy to measure. BUN can be tested before and after dialysis to see how much waste has been removed. The test to compare your BUN levels before and after dialysis measures for what's called a urea reduction ratio. Your URR should be 60% or higher to be sure you are getting enough dialysis. Some kidney doctors may even prescribe a high URR for their patients to achieve a good URR. Talk to your kidney doctor about your URR.

Another test used to measure if you're receiving adequate dialysis is kt/v (kay-tee-over-vee). Kt/v measures clearance, or "K" (urea and other waste removal) of the dialyzer. The "t" stands for time, or how long each treatment lasts, and the "v" is the volume of fluid in your blood. Your Kt/v should be 1.2 or higher to be sure you are getting enough dialysis. If you do not get enough you may feel ill. Your skin may turn yellow. You may also have itching, your feet may swell up with fluid, or you may not want to eat. You may also find it hard to sleep, have feelings of shortness of breath, or just feel very tired. Additionally, it's important to mention that you may feel depressed or your thinking may be slower. Please make sure that you discuss this with your renal team, specifically your social worker and nephrologist. The nephrologist might make changes to or add to your medicines or dialysis treatment. Getting enough dialysis will help you live long and live well. Over time, if you do not get enough dialysis, you increase your risk of death.

Preventing Infections

As a hemodialysis patient, you should learn all you can about your treatment and what you can do to stay healthy. One important area you should know about is infectious disease. These are diseases that occur when harmful bacteria get into your body's natural defenses, making it easier for you to get infections. The following sections have information on what you can do to prevent infections of your fistula, graft, and hemodialysis catheter. If you have an AV fistula or graft access, it's so important that you wash your access before your dialysis treatment. There should be sinks at your dialysis clinic for patients to wash their access before treatment. If you are unsure how to wash your access, ask your nurse or technician, who should be happy to show you. Wash your access every day, even at home, with antibacterial soap. It's very important that you do not scratch your access. Your fingernails could be a source of infection. And most importantly, do not touch the skin after it has been cleaned for dialysis. Also, you should wear a glove if you are holding your own access site after the needles are pulled. If you have a hemodialysis catheter in your neck, be sure your hemodialysis catheter has a clean dressing every treatment. When the staff change your dressing, you should wear a mask or turn your head away and do not talk. It is important to monitor the skin around the catheter. If the area around your catheter is sore, report this to the staff. Do not shower or swim if you have a hemodialysis catheter. It is important to keep the dressing dry and in place.

Your Support System

Your support system consists of the renal team plus others who support you in your community. Collectively, this is generally called your support system. They are the people who care about you and how you are doing. They are there to assist you when you need them. They should teach you:

1. The mechanics of dialysis
2. How to manage your renal diet
3. How to cope with the various insurance forms and dialysis procedures

Your support system should offer guidance and counseling when you are afraid and feeling alone. They should offer encouragement during the ups and downs of your care. And most of all, they should teach and guide you so that you will be able to fit dialysis into your life as a part of your ongoing activities with your family and friends. Your support system should try to assist you to cope with problems and offer alternative approaches to you when appropriate. Do not hesitate to reach out to the renal team when you need them. However, your greatest support may come from your family, friends, church, and neighbors. You are a part of their life, and they are a part of yours. Do not block them out. They can help you when you need them.

Chapter 3

Your First Day at Outpatient Hemodialysis

What to Expect

Being diagnosed with kidney failure can be frightening at first; it's natural to be nervous or even apprehensive, especially on the first day of outpatient dialysis. Even if you do your research before beginning outpatient dialysis treatment, during the first visit, you will be attending a new place for several hours and meeting the renal team and other patients at the clinic. In addition, you will experience a new environment and a medical procedure that's different from what you initially received in the hospital. This new normal can be very scary and overwhelming. Educating yourself on what you can generally expect at dialysis treatment may help you relax and feel better about your first day.

On arrival at your first day of outpatient dialysis, you should be greeted by a receptionist, who should inform either the administrator, charge nurse, or social worker of your arrival. Before you begin treatment, you will have to go over and sign your admission packet to include your consent and insurance forms. Make sure you bring your insurance card and a valid form of government issued identification (driver's license, state ID, or passport) so a copy can be made. If there are any questions you want to ask about the admission process and/or forms you are completing to the dialysis clinic, the healthcare team, or the dialysis process, this would be a good time to ask these questions. Once you have completed filling out the admission packet and insurance forms, your nurse or technician should be ready to bring you back into the clinic to prepare you for dialysis treatment.

What to Bring and Wear to the Dialysis Clinic

Normally, on the days you have dialysis, you will be sitting in a dialysis chair anywhere from three to four hours per session, so you'll want to be as comfortable as possible. Wear something comfortable that you don't mind getting blood on, if that should happen. During my career, many patients used to complain of being cold from the facility air conditioner. The facility may be chilly, and during dialysis your blood is circulating outside your body. For this reason, you may want to bring warm socks, a sweatshirt or sweater, and maybe a hat to help you keep warm and comfortable. If you have a hemodialysis catheter in your chest, be sure to wear a shirt that opens in the front. Also, remember where your dialysis access is located. If you have a graft or fistula on your arm, be sure your sleeves are loose enough to roll up.

In addition to warm clothes, you may want to bring a book, crossword puzzle, laptop, or music device. Most outpatient centers have televisions, so make sure you bring headphones with you to hear the sound. See if the facility has an internet connection or Wi-Fi, so you can browse online while at dialysis treatment.

Before Your Treatment Starts

Once your dialysis nurse or technician greets you, they will show you how to obtain your weight before each treatment. Then your nurse or technician should show you how to wash your vascular access until you know how to perform this task yourself. After washing and cleaning your access, you will be escorted to your dialysis chair. At this time, your dialysis nurse obtains your vital signs pre-dialysis treatment to include your standing and sitting blood pressure, temperature, and pulse rate. The nurse should come by soon to check your heart rate, listen to your lungs for the presence of fluid, and check your ankles for edema (fluid). At this time, most patients are unpacking their belongings, such as their blankets, pillows, or headphones, and getting settled into the chair for treatment. The dialysis chairs recline, and there is a table tray on each side of the chair to lay items on.

Your Hemodialysis Treatment

Finally, it's time to begin your first outpatient dialysis treatment. You may be anxious at this moment, but know that it's going to be okay. Thousands of people have traveled this road before you.

At this time, your dialysis nurse will begin to prepare your access for needle placement. If you have an AV fistula or graft in your arm, it will be wiped with an antibacterial solution to kill any bacteria on your arm. (This is usually done with an alcohol or betadine solution.) Once both needles are placed in your access, you may be given heparin (a blood thinner) to keep your blood from clotting in the tubing during dialysis treatment. The arterial needle, one of the two needles placed in your access, will carry your blood through the blood tubing to the dialyzer (artificial kidney) while the venous (second needle) will return the clean blood back to your body.

Chapter 3: Your First Day at Outpatient Hemodialysis

Some patients ask their kidney doctor for a numbing medicine (prescription) to be applied to the graft or AV fistula site. This numbing medicine is usually applied on the access arm forty-five minutes before their dialysis treatment. The medication is used to prevent patients from feeling the needle being inserted into their access. If you are afraid of needles, ask your kidney doctor for this prescription. Many patients get used to the needle sticks and are not bothered by them after some time.

If you have a hemodialysis catheter in your chest, the dialysis tubing will be connected to your catheter to start treatment. Once you are connected to the dialysis machine, your treatment has started. The machine will move your blood through the tubing and dialyzer (artificial kidney) to be cleaned and then returned to your body. Most patients' dialysis treatments last anywhere from three to four hours, three times per week. The blood will go through the artificial kidney fifteen to twenty times, and surprisingly, only about one to two cups of your blood will be outside your body at any given time.

Generally, you should not feel any pain or discomfort during your dialysis treatment. However, let your nurse know right away if you feel dizzy or experience any cramping during treatment. In addition, dizziness, nausea, and muscle cramps are potential side effects of low blood pressure, which could happen anytime during treatment if too much fluid is removed from you too fast. In order to avoid this, try to avoid gaining too much fluid between treatments. Removing too much fluid during treatment can contribute to low blood pressure and cramping.

During your treatment, you may notice the sound of alarms ringing from the dialysis machine from time to time. The dialysis machine continuously monitors the pressures created by your blood inside the blood tubing and dialyzer. The dialysis machine also monitors your blood pressure, blood flow rate, treatment time, the mixture and temperature of your dialysis bath, and the solution inside the dialysate that cleans your blood. If any of these measurements go outside their range, the dialysis machine sounds to alert the dialysis nurse.

When Treatment Ends

The end of dialysis treatment is the time many kidney patients look forward to. Many patients know this time by the distinct sound of the dialysis machine alarm when treatment is completed. When your dialysis treatment is completed, the nurse will return your blood through the tubing with normal saline. At this time the nurse will remove the needles from your access. Once the needles are removed pressure must be applied to your access site with a gloved hand and gauze to stop the bleeding.

Once the bleeding has stopped, a bandage or dressing with tape will be applied to your access. After the bleeding stops, the nurse should take your post-dialysis treatment vital signs to include blood pressure (sitting and standing), temperature, and pulse. In addition, your nurse should perform a post assessment to include listening to your lung and heart sounds.

Finally, you are ready to get your post-dialysis weight. The post-treatment weight will be used in the next treatment to help determine how much fluid you gained between treatments. After getting your post-dialysis weight, you are free to leave. However, if you experience any unexpected bleeding leaving the clinic or at home, immediately apply pressure to your site and either call 911 or your dialysis center.

Chapter 4

Patients Rights and Responsibilities

According to Medicare, patients with end-stage kidney disease have certain rights and responsibilities. When you report to your treatment center, ask for a copy of your rights and responsibilities to help you know what to expect from your healthcare team and what they can expect from you.

Your dialysis center may have a list that's similar to the following:

Your Rights:

- I have the right to be told about my rights and responsibilities.
- I have the right to privacy. My medical records can't be shared with anyone unless I say so.
- I have the right to be treated with respect.
- I have the right to meet with my whole renal team to plan my treatment.

- I have the right to see the dietitian for help with food planning and the social worker for counseling.
- I have the right to be told about my health in a way that I understand.
- I have the right to be told about and to choose my treatment option.
- I have the right to be told about any tests ordered for me and the test results.
- I have the right to be told about the services offered at the center.
- I have the right to be told about the process of dialysis and dialyzer reuse.
- I have the right to be told about any expenses that I have to pay for if they are not covered by insurance or Medicare.
- I have the right to be told about any financial help available to me.
- I have the right to accept or refuse any treatment or medicine my doctor orders for me.
- I have the right to be told about the rules at the treatment center (for example, rules for visitors, eating, personal conduct).
- I have the right to choose if I want to be part of any research studies.

Your Responsibilities

- I need to treat other patients and staff as I would like to be treated: with respect.
- I need to pay my bills on time. If this is hard for me, I can ask about a payment plan.
- I need to tell my renal team if I refuse any treatment or medicine that my doctor has ordered for me.
- I need to tell my renal team if I don't understand my medical condition or treatment plan.
- I need to be on time for my treatments or when I see my doctor.
- I need to tell the staff at the center if I know that I'm going to be late or miss a treatment or visit with my doctor.
- I need to tell my renal team if I have medical problems, am going to the dentist, am being seen/treated by another doctor, or have recently been to the hospital.
- I need to follow the rules at the center.
- I need to get to and from the center for my treatments. I can talk with my social worker if I need help doing this. Medicare doesn't pay for transportation.

Chapter 5
Understanding Patient Grievance Policy

Federal regulations require kidney dialysis centers to ensure that dialysis patients are aware of their rights and responsibilities. The education must include the patients rights to file a grievance. To help patients with this process, there are ESRD (End Stage Renal Disease) networks set up across the United States and U.S. territories. The ESRD Network consists of Medicare-approved facilities in designated geographic areas specified by Medicare. Dialysis and transplant providers in the ESRD network caring for ESRD patients coordinate patient referrals and access to resources in a more efficient manner. The ESRD network acts as the administrative governing body to this network of providers and is a liaison to the federal government. To help achieve coordinated delivery of ESRD services, representatives of hospitals and health facilities serving dialysis and transplant patients in each area of the country are linked with patients, physicians, nurses, social workers, dietitians, and technicians in the network. The ESRD network can help dialysis patients with concerns about their care. If you have a concern, the network's role is to serve as an investigator, facilitator, referral agent, coordinator, and/or educator. The role of the network in a grievance is to:

- Keep communications open between patients and ESRD facility staff on issues, problems, or grievances
- Ensure problems are solved as quickly as possible
- Help patients feel comfortable taking their concerns to an appropriate authority without fear of mistreatment or retaliation
- Help patients through the grievance process

If you have a concern about the treatment you are receiving at your dialysis clinic, first try to speak with the facility social worker, director of nursing, or administration about your concern. The dialysis facility should have the steps for its grievance procedures posted usually in the patient waiting area. You are encouraged to allow the facility to address the issue first. However, this is not a requirement. Usually the network will become involved if:

- You are not comfortable handling the issue at the facility level first.
- You believe your concerns were not resolved at the facility level.

If you would like someone else to represent you in a situation where you don't feel comfortable doing so, you may appoint a representative to help explain the problem. You may choose anyone you wish as long as the individual that represents you has your authorization to process the grievance on your behalf.

In some circumstances, the grievance may be reported to the state survey agency. This agency inspects dialysis facilities. In issues of "immediate jeopardy" or life-threatening situations, the state agency has the authority to shut down a facility until it is safe. If you need to contact your ESRD network, ask your clinic social worker for the information. The network will investigate grievances received by phone, by fax, by email, or in writing.

What Is the Time Frame for Grievances?

Usually, there is a time frame for grievances to be processed. Each network may have a different time frame, so be sure to check with your network on their time frame for processing grievances. Below is an outline of the usual grievance time frame.

- Network staff will determine the appropriate method for processing a grievance. Most grievances can be resolved in less than five days.
- The network staff will notify the grievant by mail or email on the next business day, if a case is referred to another agency.
- The more serious cases may be required to go through a quality case review. In these situations, medical records are requested, and staff, patients, and other provider records may be reviewed. The patient's written consent may be required.
- Usually, every effort is made to complete all investigations within sixty days. If the case is not closed within sixty days, all parties will be advised of the delay and when it is expected to conclude.
- The patient or his/her representative will be advised of whom to contact if not satisfied with the network's processing of the grievance.
- Usually, a follow-up contact will be made to you at the conclusion of the investigation. This contact is to determine your level of satisfaction with the grievance process. Your participation is voluntary.

Chapter 6

Treatment Options for Kidney Failure: Hemodialysis and Peritoneal Dialysis

Developing kidney failure means that you have some decisions to make about your medical treatment. If you choose to receive treatment, your choices are hemodialysis, peritoneal dialysis, and kidney transplantation. In this chapter, we'll focus on the first two, and we'll explore transplantation in the following chapter.

Each option has advantages and disadvantages. You may also choose to forgo treatment. By learning about your choices, you can work with your doctor to decide what's best for you. No matter which treatment you choose, you'll need to make some changes in your life, including how you eat and plan your activities. With the help of this guide, your doctor, renal team, family, and friends, you can lead a full and active life.

Hemodialysis

Hemodialysis is the use of a machine to clean wastes from the blood after the kidneys have failed. The blood travels through tubes to a dialyzer (artificial kidney), which removes wastes and extra fluid. The cleaned blood then flows through another set of tubes back into the body. Hemodialysis is usually done in a dialysis center by trained nurses and technicians. This type of treatment is done three times per week and usually lasts three to four hours per treatment. Hemodialysis can also be done at home with the help of a partner, usually a family member or friend. If you decide to do home hemodialysis, you and your caregiver will receive special training.

Home Hemodialysis

There are many patients on hemodialysis that perform hemodialysis at home. This is done with a small hemodialysis machine given to patients to use at home by the dialysis facility. The machine operates like those at the dialysis center, but is smaller and easy to use. Most patients have someone who helps them do home dialysis. However, some people do the process themselves. Most patients who do home dialysis do four to five treatments a week. Generally, a typical day of doing home hemodialysis may look like this. You would set up and prepare the dialysis, which takes about fifteen to thirty minutes. Then you would weigh yourself and obtain your vital signs to include blood pressure, pulse, and temperature. Get comfortable in your chair or bed to begin your treatment. You would then either connect the machine to your access. Some patients have their trained helper insert the needles into their arms, or they do it themselves. Once you're hooked up to the machine, you can spend your treatment time watching TV, reading, surfing the net, doing a crossword puzzle, or sleeping. After you finish your treatment, your helper or you would disconnect you from the machine and remove your needles. It takes about fifteen to twenty minutes to clean up from treatment. In addition, you have to fill out some paperwork recording your treatment. To do home hemodialysis, you'll need a way for the machine to access your blood. There are three kinds of access: a Central Venous Catheter (CVC), an AV fistula, and an AV graft. A CVC is usually a temporary access port. A fistula or graft is a permanent access placed below the skin. A small surgery is needed to have a fistula or graft placed. The surgery is usually in and out, and you can go home the same day.

Home Hemodialysis Considerations and Benefits

If you decide to do home hemodialysis, like with all medical treatments, there are some things to consider. If you need a helper with your treatments, it should be someone that you trust and rely on. This person should have good vision and steady hands. Home hemodialysis routinely requires needles. You or your helper should be comfortable inserting the needles. You will receive home hemodialysis training from your dialysis center. In addition, you will need a comfortable place to perform your regular treatments and somewhere to store your supplies. You will also need a standard electrical outlet and a faucet or under sink connection. This is a requirement to operate the dialysis machine.

Benefits of Home Hemodialysis

There are many benefits to home hemodialysis:

- You can do dialysis in the comfort and privacy of your home.
- You don't need to travel to the dialysis center every day. You'll usually visit the clinic once or twice a month to visit your medical team.
- You may have fewer diet restrictions than with other dialysis options.

- You can travel with your home hemodialysis machine, making vacations more easier to manage.

- Frequent home dialysis treatments can remove excess fluid more gently.

If you think home hemodialysis is something you may be interested in, talk with your kidney doctor about which treatment option is right for you. Remember, home dialysis is just one of the many treatment options for kidney failure.

Peritoneal Dialysis

Peritoneal dialysis is another procedure that removes extra water, balances electrolytes, and removes wastes from your body. This type of dialysis uses the lining of your abdomen to filter your blood. The lining is called the peritoneal membranes and acts as the artificial kidney.

This is how peritoneal dialysis works. A mixture of minerals and sugar dissolved in water, called a dialysis solution, travels through the soft tube into your abdomen. The sugar, called dextrose, draws wastes, chemicals, and extra water from the tiny blood vessels in your peritoneal membrane into the dialyzer solutions. After several hours, the used solution is drained from your abdomen through the tube, taking the wastes from your blood with it. Then you fill your abdomen with a fresh dialysis solution, and the cycle is repeated. Each cycle is called an exchange.

Before starting peritoneal dialysis, a surgeon places a small, soft tube called a catheter into your abdomen. The catheter tends to work better if there is adequate time for healing—usually ten days to three weeks for the insertion site to heal. This is another way in which planning your dialysis access can improve treatment success. This catheter stays there permanently to help transport the dialysis solution to and from your abdomen.

There are three types of peritoneal dialysis:

Continuous Ambulatory Peritoneal Dialysis (CAPD) is the most common type of peritoneal dialysis. It requires no machine and can be done in any clean, well-lit place. With CAPD, your blood is always being cleaned. The dialysis solution passes from a plastic bag through the catheter and into your abdomen, where it stays for several hours with the catheter sealed. The period that dialysis solution is in your abdomen is called the dwell time. Next, you drain the dialysis back into the bag for disposal. You then use the same catheter to refill your abdomen with fresh dialysis solution so the cleaning process can begin again. With

CAPD, the dialysis solution stays in your abdomen for a dwell time of four to six hours (or more). The process of draining the used dialysis solution and replacing it with a fresh solution takes about thirty to forty minutes. Most people change the dialysis solution at least four times a day and sleep with solution in their abdomen at night. Also, with CAPD, it's not necessary to wake up and perform dialysis tasks during the night.

Continuous Cycler-Assisted Peritoneal Dialysis (CCPD) uses a machine called a cycler to fill and empty your abdomen three to five times during the night while you sleep. In the morning, you begin one exchange with a dwell time that lasts the entire day. You may do an additional exchange in the middle of the afternoon without the cycler to increase the amount of waste removed and to reduce the amount of fluid left behind in your body.

If you weigh more than 175 pounds, or if your peritoneum filters waste slowly, you may need a combination of CAPD and CCPD to get the right dialysis dose. For example, some people use a cycler at night but also perform one exchange during the day. Others do four exchanges during the night. You will work with your renal team to determine the best schedule for you.

Both types of peritoneal dialysis are usually performed by the patient without help from a partner. CAPD is a form of self-treatment that needs no machine. However, with CCPD, you need a machine to drain and refill your abdomen. The most common problem with peritoneal dialysis is peritonitis, a serious abdominal infection. This infection can occur if the opening where the catheter enters your body becomes infected or if contamination occurs as the catheter is connected/disconnected from the bags. Peritonitis requires antibiotics treatment by your doctor. Peritoneal dialysis procedures must be strictly followed in order to avoid peritonitis, and it's important to learn to recognize the early signs, which include fever, unusual color or cloudiness of the used fluid, and redness or pain around the catheter. If you experience any of these signs, immediately report them to your doctor so that peritonitis can be treated quickly to avoid serious health problems.

Dialysis Is Not a Cure

Hemodialysis and peritoneal dialysis are treatments that help replace the work your kidneys did. These treatments help you feel better and live longer, but they don't cure kidney failure. Although patients with kidney failure are now living longer than ever, over the years, kidney disease can cause problems such as heart disease, bone disease, arthritis, nerve damage, infertility, and malnutrition. These problems won't go away with dialysis, but doctors now have new and better ways to prevent or treat them. If you experience any of these complications, report them to your kidney doctor.

Refusing or Withdrawing Treatment

For many people, dialysis not only extends life but also improves quality of life. For others who have serious ailments in addition to kidney failure, dialysis may seem a burden that only prolongs suffering. You have the right to refuse or withdraw from dialysis if you feel you have no hope of leading a life with dignity and meaning. You may want to speak with your spouse, family, religious counselor, or social worker as you make this decision. If you withdraw from dialysis treatment or refuse to begin, then you may live for a few days or several weeks, depending on your health and your remaining kidney function. Your doctor can give you medicine to make you more comfortable during this period. Should you change your mind about refusing dialysis, you may start or resume your treatments at any time.

Even if you are satisfied with your quality of life on dialysis, you should think about circumstances that might make you want to stop dialysis treatment. At some point in a medical crisis, you might lose the ability to express your wishes to your doctor. An advance directive is a statement or document in which you give instructions either to withhold treatment or to provide it, depending on your wishes and the specific circumstances. An advance directive may be a living will—a document that details the conditions under which you would want to refuse treatment. You may state that you want your healthcare team to use all available means to sustain your life, or you may specify that you want to be withdrawn from dialysis if you become permanently unresponsive or fall into a coma from which you won't wake up. In addition to dialysis, other life-sustaining treatments that you may choose or refuse include:

- Cardiopulmonary resuscitation (CPR)
- Tube feeding
- Mechanical/artificial respiration (ventilator or extracorporeal membrane oxygenation (ECMO))
- Tracheostomy
- Antibiotics

Chapter 6: Treatment Options for Kidney Failure

- Surgery
- Blood transfusion

Another form of advance directive is called a durable power of attorney for healthcare decisions or a healthcare proxy. In this type of advance directive, you assign a person to make healthcare decisions for you if you become unable to make them for yourself. Make sure the person you name understands your values and is willing to follow through on your instructions. Each state has its own laws governing advance directives. You can obtain an advance directive from your social worker.

Chapter 7

Treatment Options for Kidney Failure: Kidney Transplants

Yet another form of treatment for kidney failure is kidney transplantation. This is a procedure that involves surgically placing a functioning kidney or kidneys (e.g., pediatric en bloc or dual kidney transplant) from another person into your body. The donated kidney/kidneys does the work that your failed kidney/kidneys used to do.

What Is a Transplant Evaluation?

If you decide that a kidney transplant is right for you, discuss your decision with your kidney doctor. First, you must be evaluated before being considered for a kidney transplant. The transplant evaluation is a process where you are closely examined to see if your body can handle the kidney transplant surgery safely and whether you have an adequate caregiver/support system to help you with the pre- and post-transplant course. During the transplant evaluation, you will meet with the transplant surgeon, transplant nephrologist, kidney transplant coordinator, a social worker, and a financial coordinator to discuss the pre- and post- kidney transplant stages. All of the following are normally included:

A physical exam	Genitourinary tract assessment
Cardiac screening	Pulmonary assessment
EKG	Infection assessment
Blood tests	Dental exam
Drug screening	
Cancer screening	
Psychological evaluation	
Chest X-ray	
Insurance/financial evaluation	

For you to be a kidney transplant candidate, you must have a reasonably healthy heart and lungs and should not have conditions that could shorten your life. You must not have an active infection, unstable heart disease, or other severe medical problems that would put you in danger during a major operation. Active cancer is the only absolute contraindication. A candidate's age is not as important as their state of health, but each transplant center varies with regard to age and other factors that would exclude you from receiving a kidney transplant from their center. Be sure to check around.

What Is a Waiting List?

After you are evaluated and approved, you will be immediately added to a list of other candidates waiting to receive a kidney transplant. Your name will be added to the United Network of Organ Sharing (UNOS) and to a transplant resource center in your state. UNOS has eleven regions divided into sixty-two local areas. Kidneys are usually distributed locally first, then regionally, and last nationally. You may get on multiple regional lists and fly to the area where the kidney is.

While you are on the waiting list, it is important to update the transplant center of any changes in your health. You will also be required to send in blood samples, often called sera, to the transplant center at the center's desired frequency. These blood samples help to readily run tests such as HLA (tissue) to see how well matched your HLA (tissue) is to the potential deceased donor HLA when you get a deceased donor kidney offer. In addition, it provides an ongoing analysis to see if you have preformed antibodies that can be a result of a miscarriage/pregnancy, blood transfusions, infections, and minor surgical or dental procedures while waiting on the list. Vital to getting that exciting phone call, it is important to notify the transplant center if you move or change telephone numbers. The center will need to get a hold of you immediately when a kidney/kidneys become available.

Kidney Transplant Operation: How Does It Work?

If you have a living donor, you will schedule the operation in advance. You and your donor will be operated on at the same time, usually in side-by-side rooms. One team of surgeons will perform the nephrectomy—the removal of the kidney from the donor, while another prepares the recipient for placement of the donated kidney. If you are on a waiting list for a deceased donor kidney, you must be ready to hurry to the hospital as soon as a kidney becomes available. Once there, you will give a blood sample for the antibody cross-match test. A surgeon places the new kidney/kidneys inside your lower abdomen and connects the artery and vein of the new kidney/kidneys to your artery and vein. Your blood flows through the donated kidney/kidneys, which makes urine, just like your own kidneys did when they were healthy. The new kidney/kidneys may start working right away or may take up to a few weeks to make urine. Unless your own kidneys are causing infection or high blood pressure, they are left in your body and not removed.

Preparation for a Kidney Transplant

The transplantation process has many steps. However, you'll want to talk with your doctor first before making this decision because transplantation isn't for everyone. Your doctor may tell you that you have a condition that would make transplantation dangerous or unlikely to succeed. You may receive a kidney from a member of your family (living, related donor), from a person who has recently died (deceased donor or a directed deceased donor), or sometimes from a spouse or a very close friend (living, unrelated donor). If you don't have a living donor, you are placed on a waiting list for a deceased donor kidney. The wait for a deceased donor kidney can take many years depending mostly on your blood type. The transplant team considers four factors in matching kidneys with potential recipients. These factors help predict whether your body's immune system will accept the new kidney or reject it.

- **Blood type:** Your blood type (A, B, AB, or O) must be compatible with the donor's. This is the most important matching factor.

- **Human leukocyte antigen (HLAs):** Your cells carry six important HLAs, three inherited from each parent. Family members are most likely to have a complete match. You may still receive a kidney if the HLAs aren't a complete match as long as your blood type matches the organ donors and other tests are negative.

- **Panel reactive antibodies (PRA):** This blood test determines if you already have any specific antibodies and would therefore be "sensitized" (an acute rejection response) to any antigens of HLA from a potential kidney donor.

- **Cross-matching antigen:** The last test before implanting an organ is the cross-match. A small sample of your blood will be mixed with a sample of the organ donor's blood in a tube to see if there's a reaction. If no reaction occurs, the result is called a negative cross-match, and the transplant operation can proceed.

How Long Does a Kidney Transplant Take?

How long you'll have to wait for a kidney depends on many things, but it's primarily determined by the availability of donors with a compatible blood type and the degree of matching between you and the

Chapter 7: Treatment Options for Kidney Failure

donor. Some people wait several years for a good match, while others get matched within a few months. There aren't enough deceased donors for every person who needs a transplant, and you must be placed on a waiting list. However, if a voluntary donor wants to give you a kidney, the transplant can be scheduled as soon as you are both evaluated and cleared to move forward with surgery. Check with your transplant center since we are in a post COVID-19 world now. Avoiding the long wait is a major advantage of having a donation.

The surgery usually takes three to four hours, or it could take longer if the surgeon experiences any problems during the surgery. The usual hospital stay is about four to five days. After you leave the hospital, you will have regular follow-up visits at the transplant center. If a living donor has given you a kidney, a new technique for removing a kidney uses a smaller incision and may make it possible for the donor to leave the hospital in two to three days, depending on the recovery process. Statistically, between 85% and 90% of transplants from deceased donors are working one year after surgery. Transplants from living donors, whether a blood relative or unrelated, tend to last longer than transplants from deceased donors.

Post-Kidney Transplant Care

As with any major surgery, you will probably feel sore and groggy when you wake up. However, many transplant recipients report feeling much better immediately after surgery. Some transplanted kidneys even take a few weeks to start working (called "sleepy kidney"), and you might need to continue hemodialysis for a few more weeks until the kidney/kidneys "wake up." Even if you wake up feeling great, you will need to stay in the hospital for up to a week to recover from surgery, and longer if you have any complications. Your body's immune system is designed to keep you healthy by sensing "foreign invaders," such as bacteria, and reject them. But your immune system will also sense that your new kidney is foreign. To keep your body from rejecting it, you will have to take drugs that turn down, or suppress, your immune response. You may have to take two or more of these rejection-preventing medicines (immunosuppressants), as well as other medications, to treat or prevent other health problems. Your kidney transplant team will help you learn what each pill is for and when to take it. Be sure that you understand the instructions for taking your medicines before you leave the hospital.

If you have been on hemodialysis, you will find that your post transplant diet is less restrictive. You can drink more fluids and will likely be able to eat many of the fruits and vegetables you were previously told to avoid. You may even need to gain a little weight, but be careful not to gain too much weight too quickly, and avoid salty foods that can lead to high blood pressure. Work with your dietitian to make sure you are following a healthy eating plan.

Possible Kidney Transplant Complications

Transplant is the closest thing to a cure, but no matter how good the match, your body may reject your new kidney. The doctor will prescribe immunosuppressants to help prevent your body's immune system from attacking the kidney, a process called rejection. A common cause of rejection is not taking the rejection-preventing medication as prescribed. You will need to take immunosuppressants every day for as long as the transplanted kidney is functioning. However, sometimes even these drugs can't stop your body from rejecting the new kidney. If this happens, the transplant doctors will make every attempt to save the transplanted kidney/kidneys with stronger medicines and/or rehospitalization to treat the rejection.

Despite all the transplant team's efforts, there is still a chance that you might end back on some form of dialysis and possibly wait for another transplant. You can help prevent rejection by taking your medicines, following your diet, and watching closely for signs of rejection, like fever or soreness in the area of the new kidney or a change in your urine (lots of bubbles or a decrease in the amount). Report any such changes to your kidney transplant team as soon as possible. Immunosuppressants can weaken your immune system, which can lead to infections (viral, fungal, or bacterial). Some of the medications the doctor will prescribe to you after transplant are to prevent complications from infections. Some of the rejection-preventing medicines that the kidney transplant doctor can prescribe may also change your appearance, possibly causing your face to get fuller, development of acne or facial hair, or even some hair loss. Diet and makeup can help, however, and not all patients have these medication side effects.

Immunosuppressants work by diminishing the ability of immune cells to function. In some patients, over long periods of time, this diminished immunity can increase the risk of developing cancer. Some immunosuppressants cause cataracts, diabetes, high blood pressure, and bone disease. When used over time, these drugs may also cause liver or kidney damage in a few patients. Even if you do everything you're supposed to do, your body may still reject the new kidney, or you may have an infectious or cancer transplant related complication that you may need to return to dialysis. Unless your kidney transplant team determines that you are no longer a good candidate for transplantation, you can go back on the waiting list for another kidney.

Diet for Transplantation

Diet for transplant patients is less limited than it is for dialysis patients. Although you may still have to cut back on some foods, your diet will probably change as your medicines, blood values, weight, and blood pressure change. You may need to count calories as your medicine may give you a bigger appetite and cause you to gain weight. Also, you may have to eat less salt; your medication may cause your body to retain sodium, leading to high blood pressure.

Pros and Cons of Kidney Transplants

Pros:

- A transplanted kidney works like a normal kidney.
- You may feel healthier or "more normal."

- You have fewer diet restrictions.
- You won't need dialysis.
- Patients who successfully go through the selection process have a higher chance of having a longer life.

Cons

- It requires major surgery.
- You may need to wait for a donor.
- Your body may reject the new kidney, so one transplant may not last a lifetime.
- You will need to take immunosuppressant medicines for the duration of your functioning kidney transplant, which may cause complications.

Communicating with Your Kidney Transplant Team

There is a lot of information to learn about transplantation, if you decide to get one. If you do decide to take this route and get on the transplant list, here are some questions you may want to ask your healthcare team:

- Is transplantation the best treatment choice for me? Why?

- What are my chances of having a successful transplant?
- How do I find out whether a family member or friend can donate?
- What are the risks to a family member or friend who donate?
- If a family member or friend doesn't donate, how do I get placed on a waiting list for a kidney? How long will I have to wait?
- What symptoms does rejection cause?
- For how long does a transplant work?
- What is expected of my caregiver/support team in the pre- and post-kidney transplant stages?
- What side effects do immunosuppressants cause?
- Who will be on my healthcare team? How can these people help me?
- Whom can I talk to about finances, sexuality, or family concerns?
- How or where can I talk to other people who have faced this decision?

Just as you have the right to refuse dialysis, you also have the right to refuse transplantation. As you make this decision, you may want to talk to your spouse, family, religious counselor, or social worker.

Chapter 8

How to Care for Your Access

What Is a Hemodialysis Vascular Access?

Hemodialysis cleans your blood through a fistula, graft, or catheter. If you have kidney failure, one of these will be your lifeline. Make sure you talk with your doctor to decide which type of vascular access is best for you. You may be asking yourself, why is a vascular access important to me? This is a good question, especially when you are first diagnosed with kidney failure. Your access is your dialysis lifeline. Some patients have only a few sites for vascular access. It is very important to care for your access so it will last as long as possible. Many patients used to ask me, what happens in vascular access surgery? What I usually say to them is that a fistula or graft is most often placed in an arm, but sometimes it can be placed in your leg as well. You and your doctor should decide which type of access will work best for you. Your doctor will ultimately decide which type of access will work best for you. However, do ask your doctor if a fistula will work for you.

Normally, surgery for a fistula or graft is often done with local anesthesia on an outpatient patient basis. Medications may be needed for mild to moderate pain. Sometimes swelling of the arm may occur for a few days or weeks. If this happens, elevate your arm on a pillow to reduce the swelling.

Once the surgery is performed, patients often ask when they can use their access. Some doctors prefer getting an access created a few months before it is needed for dialysis. If a new access is used too soon after surgery, it can be damaged. A new fistula should ideally not be used for three to four months after surgery. A new graft should not be used for three to six weeks. However, there are some accesses that can be used much sooner. Ask your surgeon for verification.

During your recovery time after surgery, if you have a fistula, exercising your arm by squeezing a tennis ball will bring more blood flow to the access so it can work more effectively. As I mentioned, squeezing a rubber ball, tennis ball, or putty several times a day for at least thirty to forty-five minutes can also help develop and mature your fistula to be used for hemodialysis dialysis.

Chapter 8: How to Care for Your Access

Vascular access is a way to reach the blood vessels for hemodialysis. There are three types:

Fistula

A fistula is your artery and vein sewed together. Blood from the artery makes the vein thicker so it can be used for hemodialysis. The vein stretches over time, allowing needles to be put in the fistula. A fistula is often the longest lasting and best access. Fistulas are the gold standard for hemodialysis.

Advantages:

- Permanent
- Beneath the skin
- Lasts the longest, up to twenty years
- Provides greater blood flow for better hemodialysis treatment
- Fewer infections and other complications
- Fewer hospitalizations

Disadvantages:

- May not mature/develop
- Not possible for all patients
- Usually cannot be used for at least six to eight weeks

AV Graft

A graft is a tube, usually made of plastic, that connects an artery to a vein together, allowing needles to be put in it. Grafts are the second best way to get access to the bloodstream for hemodialysis.

Advantages:

- Permanent
- Beneath the skin
- May be used after two weeks, in some cases
- May work in patients with poor veins

Disadvantages:

- Increased hospitalizations
- Increased risk for clotting
- Increased risk for serious infections
- Increased risk for other complications and repair procedures
- Does not last as long as a fistula

Catheter

A catheter is a plastic tube inserted into a vein in the neck, chest, or groin to provide vascular access for hemodialysis. The tip rests in your heart. It is usually a temporary access. It is the third choice for getting access to the bloodstream for hemodialysis. For some patients, it is the only choice, and it will need to be used as a permanent access. Catheters may be used for a short time while a fistula or graft is healing. However, in some patients with very poor veins and arteries, a permanent catheter may be placed in the chest.

Advantages:

- Can be used immediately after placement

Disadvantages:

- Higher infection rates, which can be very serious or fatal
- Increased hospitalizations
- Does not last long, usually less than one year
- May require longer treatment times
- Prolonged use may lead to inadequate dialysis
- Cannot shower without special appliance
- High rates of clotting, requiring frequent procedures
- Risk of destroying important vein

Three Problems to Avoid to Keep Your Access Working

In having a hemodialysis access, you can encounter many problems. Below are three problems to avoid to keep your access working for hemodialysis.

Infection

Infection is a big problem in the outpatient hemodialysis unit. You can prevent an access infection by keeping your access clean. Be sure your access is washed with antibacterial soap and iodine/alcohol prep before using it for dialysis. Also, tell the nurse if your access is warm, red, or has pus drainage, or if you have a fever. To prevent an access infection, ask your renal team how you should clean your access. Do you need to cover your access in the bathtub or shower? Can you swim in a pool or lake? Who should you call if you have an access problem?

Access Blockage

Access blockage can stop your access from working, which could prevent you from receiving dialysis. To prevent your access from blockage or clotting, learn how to feel the thrill (vibration) and listen for the bruit (buzzing) in your access. In addition, tell the nurse if your hand is cold, abnormal in color, numb, painful, or hard to move. Notify your vascular surgeon or charge nurse if your access is not working. Also, ask your vascular surgeon if, in the event your access is blocked, it can be fixed and how.

Access Injury

Avoiding injury to your dialysis access is critical in preserving and maintaining long term use of your access. In order to keep your access safe and working well, learn how needle sites are rotated on your access. Be sure the right site is used at each treatment. Do not carry heavy weight across your access. Also, avoid any pressure on your access while you sleep, avoid tight clothing, and most importantly, do not allow blood pressure or blood draws from your access arm. Questions you should ask your renal team to prevent injury to your access are:

- What is the needle rotation pattern for my access?
- How much weight can I carry safely after surgery? When can I carry more?
- Can I wear a watch or hang a purse over my access arm?
- How can I avoid sleeping on my access arm?

The Do's and Don'ts of Access Care

Proper care should be taken of your access to make sure it stays functional and to prevent infections. Below is a list of do's and don'ts to help keep your access working for years.

Fistula/Graft

- Wash your access each day—use antibacterial soap before each dialysis treatment, and wash your access at the sink provided by your facility.
- Your access should be disinfected by your dialysis nurse before needles are placed.
- Do not touch your access after it has been disinfected.
- Do not cough or sneeze on your access.
- Wear a glove if you are holding your access after the needles are removed.
- Apply gentle pressure where the needles were removed.
- When a dialysis nurse is working near your access, your nurse should wear a surgical mask or face shield.
- Be sure needles are rotated into new sites for each dialysis treatment. (Continuous sticking in the same area causes weakness in that area.)
- Blood pressure readings or blood draws should *never* be taken on your access arm (use other arm).
- Outside the dialysis facility, blood should not be taken from your access.

Chapter 8: How to Care for Your Access

Report problems with your access immediately, including these signs and symptoms of infection: swelling, redness, drainage, heat, pain, fever and chills, absence of vibration (thrill) or sound (bruit).

- Use your access site early for dialysis.
- Be careful not to bump or hit your access.
- Do not wear jewelry or tight clothing over your access location.
- Do not scratch your access. (Fingernails can cause infection.)
- Do not sleep with your access arm under your body or head.
- Do not lift heavy objects or put pressure on your access arm.
- Check the pulse (thrill) in your arm every day.

Catheter

- Be sure your catheter has a clean dressing applied during each dialysis.
- Your catheter should be checked for signs of infection at each dialysis treatment.
- Clean gloves should be used when your nurse works with your catheter.

- You and your dialysis nurse should wear a surgical mask when you are being connected to and disconnected from the dialysis machine.
- Keep your catheter dry. Do not shower or swim.
- Report problems with your access immediately, including these signs and symptoms of infection: swelling, redness, drainage, heat, pain, and fever and chills.

Chapter 9

Making Wise Food Choices

To feel your best, you need to take your medications and come to all your dialysis treatments as scheduled—*and* choose the food you eat wisely. Your dietitian should help you learn to choose the foods that will benefit you the most and teach you the ones that can harm you. Your diet prescription is matched to your body's ability to function based on your stage of chronic kidney disease and other health problems you may have. Keep this in mind, as your diet may be different from that of another dialysis patient.

Healthy kidneys clean out the body's waste through urine. When kidneys are diseased, urine output either decreases or stops. This causes waste products to build up in the blood. Dialysis removes part of these waste products. However, they still build up in your blood between treatments. Therefore, it's important to eat foods that will not cause you further harm. Listed below are common concerns that your dietitian can help you understand.

Protein

Protein is found in all animal products: meat, poultry, fish, eggs, and milk, and in smaller amounts in bread, cereals, and vegetables. Since you lose some protein during each dialysis treatment, you need to eat more protein than the average person. When the protein in your blood (called albumin) is too low, you are more likely to get sick and need to be in the hospital. It is important that you eat enough protein every day.

Here are some high-protein foods that you can include in your diet:

Food Item	Grams of Protein/Measure
• Lean meat, pork, poultry (no skin), fish	7 gm/oz
• Tuna fish (in water)	8 gm/cup
• Egg (medium-sized)	7 gm/egg

If your albumin (protein) is low and you don't feel like eating protein, you may need to use protein supplements. **(Ask your dietitian before using these products.)**

Other suggestions for increasing the protein content of your food:

1. Have an egg or an egg substitute every day for breakfast.

2. Add hard-boiled eggs or chunks of meat to salads and casseroles.
3. If you have trouble chewing meat, use ground meats for sandwiches, meatloaf, etc.
4. Don't use lunch meats, hotdogs, or bacon for protein as they are high in sodium, are highly processed, and will fill you up without giving you the protein you need. Instead, use leftover meat, chicken, tuna, or eggs to make sandwiches.
5. If you don't feel well enough to cook, ask for help! Call a family member, friend, or neighbor. Your social worker can help you find a senior center or a Meals on Wheels program that can assist you with this situation.
6. If you can't eat large meals, then have several small meals throughout the day, including a protein food each time.

Potassium

Potassium is a mineral found in many foods. However, if potassium builds up too much in your blood between dialysis treatments, it can make your heart beat irregularly or stop altogether without warning. Your dietitian should talk to you about your potassium needs, which are affected by how much urine you still make and some medications.

Phosphorus

Phosphorus is a mineral found in just about all foods, and so it cannot be totally removed from your diet. However, if you eat too much phosphorus, it can build up in your blood and cause itching and damage to your bones. To help prevent these problems, you will probably need to limit your consumption of certain foods that are high in phosphorus, such as milk products, chocolate, dried beans, and nuts. You may also need to take a medicine with your meals to grab the phosphorus from your food and "bind" it so it doesn't get into your blood. The bound phosphorus is eliminated through your stool. Some medicines used for this are calcium carbonate, Tums, Phoslo, and Renvela. These may be some of the medicines prescribed to you by the kidney doctor if your phosphorus is high. If a binder is ordered by your kidney doctor, it is important that you take it with every meal and also with snacks.

Foods that are high in phosphorus and should be limited in your diet:

- Milk and dairy products, like cheese, yogurt, ice cream, and pudding*
- Cream- or milk-based soups
- Commercial waffles and pancakes

- Chocolate
- Pepsi, Coca-Cola, and beer
- Liver
- Dried beans
- Kidney beans, pinto beans, and peas
- Oysters
- Dried fruit, including dates, figs, and raisins
- Bran cereal
- Sardines
- Nuts and seeds
- Whole wheat bread

***Limit** milk and milk products to ½ cup per day or 1 ounce of cheese each day.

The proper daily calorie intake for a hemodialysis patient is based on your ideal body weight for your height. If you are overweight, the dietician can help you plan a diet for weight loss. If you are underweight, a high-calorie plan for weight gain can be developed.

Triglycerides

Triglycerides are a type of fat that exists in your bloodstream. Excess sugar intake can increase your triglycerides. Some high triglycerides levels can cause heart disease; thus it's best to limit sugar and sweets, like cakes, cookies, pies, candy, etc. It would also be to your advantage to exercise regularly at a level you can tolerate.

Fluid Intake

Fluids are very important! To ensure an effective dialysis treatment, you should have 1,000 cc (four cups) of fluids per day. However, if you're holding too much fluid in your body, you may be told to drink less and limit your salt intake. Suitable fluids include water, ice, coffee, tea, soda, milk, juice, soup, ice cream, Jell-O, or anything that melts at room temperature.

Fluid Control

Weight Gain

Normal kidneys can control fluid balance by removing excess body fluid and putting it into urine. When the kidneys do not function well, the fluid accumulates in the body. All this excess fluid in your body and blood stream can cause high blood pressure and place a strain on the heart. Eventually, fluid collects in the lungs, making it difficult to breathe. When you first start hemodialysis the body must be brought into proper fluid balance. This is referred to as your "ideal or "goal" dry weight. As you begin to feel better, you will also begin to eat better. This may slowly add "real" weight, thereby increasing your ideal weight.

It is best to keep your fluid gain between treatments at 2-3 kilograms. You should also follow your diet paying special attention to directions concerning salt and water intake. If you find that weight gain is a repeated problem, request that the dietitian modify your diet. Excessive fluid gain is not good—it will increase your blood pressure and may cause puffy eyes or fluid buildup around your ankles. Constant excessive fluid gain places an added stress on your heart and lungs and must be avoided.

Fluid weight gain:

1. Increases blood pressure and puts extra work on the heart.
2. Results in fluid collection and swelling around the ankles.
3. Causes shortness of breath.
4. Increases weight.

Weight and blood pressure play important roles in your dialysis treatment.

Helpful Hints for Fluid Control

1. Drink only if thirsty. If you avoid high-sodium foods, you will have less thirst. Remember, foods

from restaurants and fast food establishments are generally high in salts.

2. Drink your allowed fluids with meals or medications only.

3. Try to have allowed fruits and vegetables ice cold between meals. Freeze small pieces of fruit, like grapes and strawberries.

4. Try sliced lemon wedges to produce saliva and moisten "dry" mouth or add 2 ounces of lemon juice to water and make ice.

5. Use sour hard candies/mints and chewing gum to moisten the mouth. Sugarless is more effective. Try "gator gum" or "quench" gum if available.

6. Rinse your mouth with water, but don't swallow it. Try pocket breath spray or rinsing chilled mouthwash, but don't swallow it.

7. Take medications with mealtime liquids or with applesauce, especially phosphate binders.

8. Keep in mind that you will probably be thirstier the day before dialysis than you are the day after. Avoid being in the sun and hot temperatures.

9. Measure ice allotment for the day and store in a special container in your freezer. Most people

Chapter 9: Making Wise Food Choices

find ice more satisfying than the same amount of water since it stays in the mouth longer.

10. Try to eliminate water, as it has no nourishment. Cold tea or lemonade quenches thirst better than soda, and they provide calories.

11. Use very small cups and glasses for beverages and other liquids. Any food that melts at room temperature is fluid: ice cream, sherbert, Jell-O, popsicles, fruits, and vegetables are about 90% fluid. These items should be considered liquids and should be calculated with your fluid intake.

12. Be aware that a pint (2 cups) of retained fluid equals one pound or 16 ounces of fluid gain.

13. When thirsty, try eating something like bread with margarine and jelly before taking fluids. Often, the sense of thirst is really the sensation of a dry mouth. Foods may alleviate a dry mouth.

14. Try to keep yourself as active as possible. When you are inactive, you may drink out of boredom or habit.

15. Your urinary output determines your fluid intake. If you no longer urinate, restrict fluids to 1,000 cc per day (about 4 cups or 32 ounces). If you still make urine, you may be asked to bring in a forty-

eight-hour urine collection to check your kidney function. Your doctor or dietitian will tell you how much fluid you are allowed.

16. Be sure to eat well-balanced meals, and you will have less desire for excess liquids.

17. Fluid abuse is harmful to your heart and lungs. Excess fluids must be removed by dialysis to protect you from congestive heart failure and pulmonary edema. When large amounts of fluid are removed during dialysis, muscle cramping and other unpleasant symptoms can occur.

18. Learn to control your liquid intake so that you spend less time in the hospital and avoid needing extra dialysis treatments.

Chapter 10

Additional Important Information

There are some medications you may be asked to take during dialysis or at home. The following are some of those medications:

Phosphate Binders

Tums, Phoslo, calcium carbonate, Renvela

- These pills bind with the phosphorus in the food, which then leaves the body in the stool. It is important that these pills be taken right before or during the meal, so they can work their best to prevent the body from soaking up phosphorus from the food.
- May cause constipation.

Vitamins and Supplements

- Iron - Needed for healthy red blood cells. Iron will be given to you through your dialysis blood line/tubing during your treatment.

- Folic Acid - Part of vitamin B group. It helps your body make red blood cells.
- Vitamin D - Needed to absorb calcium from food and send it to the bones.
- Multivitamins - Prevent vitamin deficiency.

Laxatives*

- Metamucil - Adds bulk to the diet to help prevent constipation. Needs to be mixed with water, so may not be good for people with fluid control problems.
- Colace - Helps prevent constipation by making the stool soft.
- Ducolax - Helps relieve constipation by making the bowels more active.
- Sorbitol - Helps relieve constipation.
- Avoid any laxative containing magnesium. (e.g., milk of magnesium)

*Important: Do not take non-prescription laxatives without checking with your doctor first.

Antibiotics

- Used to kill bacteria that cause infections. Each antibiotic attacks certain bacteria, and your doctor decides which drug is right for you.

- Many antibiotics need to be given after treatment on dialysis days. Check with your doctor.
- If you get a skin rash, funny feeling in your mouth, dizziness, ear ringing, nausea, or diarrhea while taking antibiotics, notify your doctor.

Antihypertensive (Blood Pressure Medication)

Blood pressure pills may cause a person to feel dizzy or faint when standing up. To avoid this:

- Always get up slowly.
- After lying down, get up slowly and sit on the side of the bed before standing.
- Always sit down when feeling faint.
- If faintness persists throughout the day, notify your doctor or dialysis unit.

A combination of two to three antihypertensive drugs may be used rather than a high dose of just one drug. **Please check with your kidney doctor before taking any over-the-counter medications or any medications ordered by another physician.**

What Is Blood Pressure?

Blood pressure (BP) is the amount of pressure within our arteries produced by the heart when it pumps to circulate blood through the body. Many patients normally ask, what is a normal blood pressure? A blood pressure is measured at two levels: systolic and diastolic. The systolic is the top number when the heart is contracting and pushing the blood through the arteries. The diastolic is the bottom number when the heart is relaxing between contractions. An average blood pressure is 120/80.

What Further Damage Can Result from High Blood Pressure?

Due to the abnormally high pressure, your blood vessels begin to lose their ability to stretch. Blood vessels in the brain may burst when their walls become weakened, and a "stroke" can occur. A stroke can cause various degrees of paralysis.

What Effect Does High Blood Pressure Have on the Kidneys?

The kidneys begin to suffer as the increased pressure damages the tiny arteries in these organs. Eventually the kidneys fail to filter out the waste products, and kidney failure follows.

What Are the Symptoms of High Blood Pressure?

Although headache, easy fatigue, shortness of breath, and dizziness occur with high blood pressure, there are many other disorders in which similar symptoms can occur. It is wise to have a physician examine you and determine whether your blood pressure requires treatment.

Why Is It Important to Know if You Have High BP?

High blood pressure imposes an extra burden on your heart and blood vessels. Pumping against an abnormally high blood pressure causes your heart to overwork. This abnormal strain on your heart can cause the walls of your heart to thicken.

What May Eventually Happen if Patients Refuse Treatment for High Blood Pressure?

The kidneys may fail, brain hemorrhage can occur, and the heart might simply not be able to stand the strain, leading to heart failure.

All hope is not lost, however. High blood pressure can be treated. Although there are many medicines to help you, you still have to do your part. Your doctor will more than likely give you specific medications to take, but he may also want you to:

- Maintain your ideal weight; do not allow excess fluid to accumulate within the body. If your doctor believes you should lose weight, maintain it at the level they suggest.

- Get plenty of relaxation. Don't wait until you are too exhausted before you rest. Plan breaks throughout the day.
- Avoid alcohol and tobacco.
- Settle your problems so they don't worry you and interfere with your peace of mind.
- Get adequate sleep.
- Get exercise, like walking, which is ideal for promoting relaxation.

What Is Anemia?

Anemia refers to a low red blood cell count (RBC). This results in a shortage of hemoglobin (formed in the red blood cell), which carries oxygen to all the cells in the body. Oxygen is needed by the body's cells for survival. An anemic patient may feel tired, dizzy, or lack energy. Anemia in dialysis patients is caused by many things, including:

1. Inadequate erythropoietin
2. Iron deficiency
3. Vitamin deficiency

Inadequate Erythropoietin

Erythropoietin is made by normal kidneys. It is the hormone that tells the bone marrow to make more red blood cells. A lack of erythropoietin means a shortage of red blood cells or low **hematocrit.** A desired hematocrit for dialysis patients is 32%-36%. Aranesp or Epogen is the synthetic form of erythropoietin that is given during hemodialysis. It helps your body make red blood cells. Your dietitian, nurse, or doctor checks the dose of Aranesp or Epogen monthly and makes changes as needed.

Iron Deficiency

Iron is needed to make red blood cells. Without iron, your hematocrit will drop. Without iron, you will feel tired and dizzy, and you will lack energy. You may even be short of breath. Dialysis patients lose iron with each blood draw and dialysis treatment. Hidden blood loss can also occur from hemorrhoids, ulcers, or tumors in the bowel. Taking iron helps build up iron stores that are used to make red blood cells. Most dialysis clinics check iron stores every three months during their lab draws. Iron pills are not absorbed well by dialysis patients, so when your iron stores are low, your doctor will order an intravenous iron medication. This will give your iron stores a boost and will help prevent you from becoming anemic.

Vitamin B Group Deficiency

Vitamin B12 and folic acid promote good blood cell growth. Dialysis removes these vitamins. To help prevent anemia, dialysis patients need to take a multivitamin supplement daily after dialysis. Nephrovite RX, Dialyvite RX, and Renavite RX are the names of multivitamins that are most commonly prescribed for dialysis patients.

Sex and Intimacy

For many people living with kidney disease, sex may be one of the last things on your mind. Patients are concerned with the physical demands of dialysis, the side effects of their medicines, hormone changes, blood pressure changes, and general tiredness. In addition, anemia, depression, anxiety, and other medical problems that occur with kidney failure may also cause a drop in energy and a change in interest in sex or intimacy. But to many patients, the ability to discuss sex and kidney disease is very important. Don't wait for your kidney doctor to bring up the subject. You should ask questions of him or her as well as discuss it with your primary care doctor. Don't be afraid to ask questions about your sex drive and your ability to perform. If you find yourself having problems, discuss it openly with your partner. Your attitude with each other, your closeness, and your sharing are a part of sex and sexuality.

Don't limit your trips out of the house to the doctor or to the dialysis unit. Go out socially, even though you may be tired. Simple things you used to enjoy can still be shared, and they may help you find an important part of yourself that feels like it's been missing.

Facts About the Flu Vaccine

1. Influenza is a highly contagious viral infection of the nose, throat, and lungs that ranks as one of the most severe illnesses of the winter season. Influenza is spread easily from person to person.

2. Influenza is spread through direct contact and through contact with the airborne virus, primarily when an infected person coughs or sneezes.

3. Symptoms of influenza are characterized by abrupt onset of high fever, chills, a dry cough, headache, runny nose, sore throat, and muscle and/or joint pain. Unlike other common respiratory infections, influenza can cause extreme fatigue lasting several days to weeks.

4. Although nausea, vomiting, and diarrhea sometimes occur during a flu infection, such symptoms are rarely prominent. Stomach flu is a misnomer

sometimes used to describe gastrointestinal illnesses that are actually caused by other microorganisms.

5. Influenza may lead to pneumonia, hospitalization, or even death, especially among the elderly and the high-risk groups. ESRD patients are considered high risk. An estimated 10% to 20% of the population contracts influenza annually.

6. Flu and pneumonia remain the fifth leading cause of death among the elderly, taking as many as 70,000 lives each year. It is estimated that up to 80% of deaths from the flu could be prevented with a "flu shot" (vaccination).

7. It is important to be vaccinated against influenza every year because the flu virus changes from year to year.

8. The most effective time to get the influenza vaccine is from early October to mid-November.

9. Medicare Part B pays for influenza vaccines, and a doctor's order is not required.

10. Influenza vaccine will not protect you from other respiratory infections, such as colds, bronchitis, or COVID-19.

11. A simple flu shot often turns out to be a life-saver for many frail and elderly patients. The flu shot helps avoid needless suffering and lowers medical costs that result from flu-related hospitalizations (i.e., pneumonia).

Who Should Get the Influenza Vaccine?

- People 65 years of age and older
- People with chronic disorders of the lungs and heart
- People who require regular medical follow-up or hospitalizations during the past year because of chronic diseases (such as kidney diseases, heart disease, diabetes, or blood diseases like sickle cell anemia)
- People who are less able to fight infections because of diseases or drug therapy, such as long-term steroids, radiation, or chemotherapy (for HIV, cancer, or transplants)
- Residents of nursing homes or other long-term care facilities that house anyone of any age with chronic medical conditions
- Healthcare workers, family members, and anyone else in contact with high-risk populations

- Anyone who wishes to reduce their chances of catching influenza, particularly those who provide essential community services

Is the Vaccine Safe?

You cannot get influenza from the vaccine. The vaccine is safe and effective and generally has few side effects. There may be some soreness, redness, or swelling where the shot is given. Other possible mild side effects include a headache and low-grade fever for a day after the vaccination. As with any medication, there is a small risk that serious problems, even death, could occur after getting a vaccine. However, the risks from the disease are much greater than the risks from the vaccine. The influenza vaccine may be given anytime during the influenza season if there are still cases of influenza in the community. However, for maximum protection, the vaccines should be given from October to mid-November.

Dental Work and Dialysis: How Are They Connected?

Routine dental checkups are very important in keeping your teeth and gums healthy. You are encouraged to visit your dentist regularly (every six months). Before you have any dental work done, such as teeth cleaning, root canal, pulling teeth, etc., it is recommended that you talk to your nephrologist. They will prescribe a single dose of antibiotics for you to take one hour before your dental work. The antibiotics protect you from infections that you can get from dental procedures. Routine dental checkups are recommended for patients with kidney failure.

Any type of dental work that makes gums bleed can cause bacteria in the mouth to get into the bloodstream. Once in the bloodstream, the bacteria can travel and cause blood infections, heart valve infections, or dialysis access infections. You may be asking, why are the heart valves and dialysis access most at risk for infection? That's a good question. The reason is the heart valve can become damaged over time due to high phosphorus levels, high fluids gains, high blood pressure, and treated infections. This damage to the valve can cause you to develop a "heart murmur." People with heart murmurs have a greater risk of infection from dental work. Most people on dialysis have a heart murmur. The bacteria can also travel from the gums and settle in the dialysis access, causing an access infection. This very serious infection requires hospitalization, IV antibiotics, and surgery to remove the access. Dialysis patients are more prone to infections because the immune system is responsible for fighting infections. A dialysis patient's immune system does not respond as quickly to fight infections as someone not on dialysis.

Penicillin is the most commonly and widely used antibiotic. Vancomycin is used for most people who are allergic to penicillin. Both medications are prescribed as a one-time dose to be taken one hour before each dental procedure. The renal team is concerned about and dedicated to protecting patients from serious and unwanted infections. Unfortunately, in the United States, 13% of deaths in chronic dialysis patients are due to infections. Take an active role in your health. See your dentist regularly, but make sure that you see your kidney doctor to get a prescription for antibiotics to take before any procedure.

Renal Bone Disease and You

As a dialysis patient, you should have a basic knowledge of kidney disease and the different treatments you need. Also, you should know from this guide or renal team about a few complications you might face. Now we will take a look at a complication you may not know much about: renal bone disease. It is a condition that affects almost all dialysis patients, and it causes their bones to become weak.

How Do You Know if You Have Renal Bone Disease?

When bone disease begins, there are usually no signs. However, if bone disease goes untreated, you may begin to have some of the symptoms listed below. Also, the dialysis team can detect if you have bone disease based on blood work results and bone X-rays.

Symptoms of renal bone disease include:

- Itching
- Bone pain
- Fractures
- Muscle weakness
- Joint pain

Even if you experience these symptoms, there is good news for you. If you work with your dialysis team and follow diet and medication recommendations, you can safeguard your bones. First, it is important to understand the relationship between your kidneys and your bones.

When your kidneys were healthy, your bones were protected. Healthy kidneys helped keep the proper amount of calcium and phosphorus in your blood. In other words, your calcium and phosphorus were in balance. Your bones need both of these important minerals to stay strong. Phosphorus comes into your body through the foods you eat. All foods have some phosphorus, so it's likely that you took in more phosphorus than you needed. Prior to having kidney failure, this was not a problem, since healthy kidneys removed the extra phosphorus.

When your kidney stopped working, calcium and phosphorus went out of balance. Your failed kidneys can't get rid of the extra phosphorus, so it continues to build up. In trying to balance calcium with extra phosphorus, your body pulls calcium from your bones, making them weak. Keeping phosphorus in balance is necessary for strong bones.

How Can You Keep Your Bones Healthy?

Achieving healthy bones is up to you and your dialysis team. You will do this with a combination of:

- Dialysis
- Diet
- Phosphate binders
- Calcium supplements
- Rocaltrol, Zemplar, or Hectorol

Dialysis

Your dialysis treatment will help remove some extra phosphorus, but not all. For dialysis to remove as much phosphorus as it can, you have to make two commitments:

1. Always come to your dialysis treatment as scheduled.
2. Stay for the full treatment time for each session of dialysis.

Diet

Your diet is something that you can control. A properly planned diet with your dietitian will help keep your calcium and phosphorus in balance. You may have to eat less of some foods and cut down on phosphorus (e.g., milk, cheese, cola, beans, peanut butter, whole grains, chocolate). This will prevent phosphorus from building up to an unhealthy level. Together with your dietitian, you can plan low-phosphorus meals that are both tasty and nutritious.

Phosphate Binders:

Phosphorus from foods you eat must be kept out of the bloodstream. Phosphorus binders act like a magnet to pull or bind the phosphorus while it is still in the stomach. Bound phosphorus cannot enter the blood and is passed out of the body in the stool. Remember to take your binders with your meals. Timing is very important! You may also be advised to take binders with snacks. Some commonly used phosphorus binders are Renagel, Tums, Phoslo, Calcichew, and Oscal.

Calcium Supplement

Your dialysis team may advise you to take additional calcium supplements. Some of the same medicines that you take as phosphate binders can be used as calcium supplements (e.g., Tums, Phoslo, Calcichew, Oscal). If used as calcium supplements, you may be advised to take these in between meals. Remember that you will still need to take your phosphorus binders as directed with meals to keep your phosphorus level down. If you have any questions about the timing of your medicine, speak with your dialysis team.

Rocaltrol or Zemplar

In order to keep your bones strong, you may be advised to take a special vitamin supplement (Rocaltrol or Zemplar). This is a special prescription form of vitamin D that your kidneys can no longer make. These medicines allow calcium to be absorbed into your blood and stored in your bones. Whether you are on Rocaltrol or Zemplar, it is very important to keep your phosphorus level under good control. Otherwise,

Chapter 10: Additional Important Information

these medicines will be placed on hold, and you will not be able to benefit from them.

You will feel better if you take control today. It will take some effort on your part, but paying attention to dialysis, diet, supplements, binders, lab values, and special vitamin D supplements will help you achieve and maintain healthier bones. With healthier bones, you can have a more active life. You should be able to continue your activities, spend more time with your friends and family, enjoy your hobbies, or perhaps go back to work. No matter how long you have been on dialysis, now is the time to take control for healthier bones.

Let's review what you can do to improve the health of your bones:

- Follow a low-phosphorus diet.
- Aim for a phosphorus level between 3.0-5.5 mg/dl.
- Take your phosphate binders with meals.
- Come to all of your dialysis treatments, and stay for the full time.
- Take your calcium supplements.

Chapter 11

Stay Healthy

If you are reading this page, hopefully you've had a chance to read through the entire guide. As mentioned before, this guide was created to support you and your family. I am dedicated to helping keep chronic kidney failure patients feeling their best. However, this takes not only teamwork but also a partnership where you—the most important member of the team—are willing to make the investment of your time and effort.

The payoff for all your hard work is feeling better and staying out of the hospital. I can give you and your family the information, but it is on you to take charge of your health. The bottom line is that whatever you decide to do or not to do has the greatest impact on your health. Much of the information you have read deals with the everyday things, much like putting gas in a car to keep it going. But there are also preventive healthcare measures that you need to take.

Compare it to the 3,000-mile oil change for your car that keeps the car's engine running and using gas efficiently.

Dialysis patients should see a dentist every six months (remember to get antibiotics first) and get a chest X-ray, EKG, and flu vaccine every year. Additionally, you should receive the pneumonia vaccine, according to the national guidelines. If you are forty years or older, you should have your eyes examined every two years. If you are fifty years or older, you should have a colonoscopy done every five to ten years to check for colon cancer. If you have diabetes, you should have your feet checked every year or more often, as recommended by a podiatrist. Even if you don't have diabetes, it's a good idea to have your feet checked by a podiatrist at least once due to the nerve damage that sometimes comes with kidney disease. If you have polycystic kidney disease or have been on dialysis for more than ten years, you should have a renal ultrasound every year to screen for cancer in your kidneys. If you are a woman, you should see a gynecologist once a year, and if you are over forty years old, have a mammogram every year. If you are a man fifty years or older, you should have a rectal exam done every year to check your prostate gland for cancer or enlargement.

Chapter 11: Stay Healthy

Ask your primary care doctor about scheduling these vaccines/tests if they haven't already been done. If you have any questions about your health, talk with your kidney doctor. Kidney disease takes time to get adjusted to; however, being armed with information can have you living the best life you can in spite of kidney failure.

Chapter 12

Coronavirus and Kidney Disease

The coronavirus disease 2019, or COVID-19, has made a devastating impact both in the United States and globally. In the United States alone, the coronavirus has more than 9 million reported cases and claimed more than 200,000 lives at the time of my writing this book. At this time, COVID-19 is a new disease, and health officials are still learning more about how it spreads, the severity of illness it causes, and to what extent it may spread in the United States.

While some cases of the coronavirus prove to be mild, the potential to develop serious complications should always be considered, especially for those individuals with comorbidities like diabetes or kidney disease. Individuals with serious underlying chronic medical conditions, like chronic lung disease, a serious heart condition, or a weakened immune system, seem to be at higher risk of severe illness from COVID-19. Patients with kidney disease who appear most at risk for COVID-19 are those with a kidney transplant, due to immunosuppressants, and those who undergo in-center hemodialysis treatment thrice weekly. Subsequently, as a result of patients with kidney disease having other comorbidities and being at high risk for the coronavirus, I decided to include an important section in this book on the coronavirus and kidney disease. What I hope to achieve with this chapter is to arm patients experiencing kidney failure with the information needed to feel comfortable navigating through this pandemic safely, wisely, and less fearfully.

About COVID-19

COVID-19 disease is a respiratory illness that spreads from person to person. The virus is thought to spread mainly between people who are in close contact with one another (within about six feet) through respiratory droplets produced when an infected person coughs or sneezes. It is also possible for someone to get COVID-19 by touching a surface or object that has the virus on it and then touching their own mouth, nose, or eyes.

Protecting Yourself at Dialysis Facilities and at Home

Dialysis is a life-saving therapy, and patients should not postpone treatment in fear of the virus. Dialysis

Chapter 12: Coronavirus and Kidney Disease

facilities can protect you and staff from respiratory infections, including COVID-19, by following the CDC recommendations. When you attend outpatient hemodialysis, you should expect to see the following preparations in place to address your safety and the staff's during this pandemic:

1. Signs should be posted at entrances instructing patients with fever and/or symptoms of COVID-19 to alert staff, so they can take appropriate precautions.
2. Signs should be posted about the importance of hand hygiene, respiratory hygiene, and cough etiquette to prevent the spread of illness.
3. Supplies (e.g., tissues, alcohol-based hand sanitizer, face masks, line trash cans) should be located near entrances, waiting rooms, dialysis chairs, and nursing stations to make it easy for staff and patients to maintain hand and respiratory hygiene and cough etiquette.
4. The patient waiting area should be organized to divide patients with symptoms from patients without symptoms.
5. The area for patients with symptoms should be at least six feet away from the area for patients without symptoms.

6. If you believe you have symptoms of COVID-19, immediately call your dialysis facility to report your symptoms to the charge nurse.

7. A staff member may be in the patient lobby area to screen all patients for symptoms and fever before entering the treatment floor.

8. You should expect to see all patients wearing a cloth face covering or face mask upon arrival at the clinic, regardless of their symptoms. If you do not have a face mask, the facility should provide you with one.

Home

If you receive assistance with your daily living activities from a direct-support provider, ask your direct support provider if they are experiencing any symptoms of COVID-19 or if they have been in contact with someone who has COVID-19. Tell your direct support provider to wear a mask and to wash their hands when they enter your home, before and after touching you (e.g., dressing, bathing/showering, transferring, toileting, and feeding), when handling tissues, or when changing linens or doing laundry. Learn about proper handwashing so that you are performing good hand hygiene. Clean and disinfect frequently touched objects and surfaces (e.g., counters, tabletops, doorknobs, bathroom fixtures, toilets, phones, keyboards, tablets, and bedside tables), and such equipment as wheelchairs, scooters, walkers, canes, oxygen tanks and tubing, communication boards, and other assistive devices, especially if you have other family members living with you.

Preparation for Those on Dialysis

There are some additional actions you can take if you have chronic kidney disease and are on dialysis during the COVID-19 pandemic.

- Create a plan of action in the event that you or nurse gets sick. Write a contact list of family, friends, neighbors, and local service agencies that can provide support in case you or your nurse becomes ill or unavailable.

- Plan at least two ways of communicating from home and work that can be used rapidly in an emergency (e.g., landline phone, cell phone, text messaging, email). Write down this information and keep it with you.

- Stock enough household items and groceries so that you will be comfortable staying home for a few weeks, or stock at least a thirty-day supply of over-the-counter and prescription medicines and any medical equipment or supplies that you might need. Some health plans allow for a ninety-day refill on prescription medications. Consider discussing this option with your healthcare provider. Make a photocopy of prescriptions, as this may help in obtaining medications in an emergency situation.

- Do not miss your dialysis treatment.
- Contact your dialysis clinic or nephrologist if you start to feel sick or have health concerns, whether they're related to COVID-19 or not.

If You Have to Venture Into the Public

It is strongly encouraged that you avoid venturing into public during the COVID-19 crisis. I already covered that COVID-19 is extremely contagious and is transmitted easily from person to person by respiratory droplets that are spread when an infected person sneezes, coughs, or talks. If you have to venture into a public setting for essentials or for dialysis treatment, the following are the CDC's protective guidelines that you should know and follow:

- Maintain a six-foot distance from others in public settings.
- Wear a cloth face covering or face mask.

- Wash hands often and thoroughly with soap and water for at least twenty seconds.
- Practice good food hygiene.

Prevention and Treatment

Currently, there is neither a vaccine nor a specific antiviral treatment to protect against or treat COVID-19. The best way to prevent infection is to take everyday preventive actions, like avoiding close contact with people who are sick and washing your hands often. Most importantly, wearing a face mask as per public health guidelines is vital until a vaccine becomes available. People with COVID-19 can seek medical care to help manage symptoms.

Getting a flu vaccine during the flu season is more important now than ever because of the ongoing COVID-19 pandemic. Flu vaccination is especially important for people who are at high risk for flu, many of whom are also at high risk for COVID-19. There is rapidly evolving information emerging about COVID-19; however, by practicing CDC recommended guidelines, you can reduce your chances significantly of getting COVID-19.

Acknowledgments

Writing a book to help patients with kidney failure was the last thing I thought I would be doing after sustaining a personal injury that ended my career. However, sitting down to research and create my thoughts has been challenging, but very rewarding. I wouldn't have ever imagined in 1985, when I entered the dialysis field as a dialysis technician, that I would one day be writing a book to assist a population of people affected by kidney disease—the ninth leading cause of death in the United States. This new role as an author is not taken lightly. As the saying goes, "To whom much is given, much will be required," and I intend to educate and spread kidney disease awareness until my final days.

With that being said, I would like to thank God, the creator of the universe, for giving me the insight, intuition, and instructions to create and write this much-needed book.

To my family—Mom, Dad, Tyisha, Cyniah, Aaron, Alicia, Takala, and Deon—I am eternally grateful to you for all your love, support, understanding, and patience throughout these years. I know I haven't been the most attentive son, father, uncle, and grandfather that I could have been; my work and advocacy has definitely been the driving force in my life, and I know family time has been sacrificed at my passion's expense. But my wish and hope is that this book shows you my dedication, compassion, and love for this work. I love you.

Allison, this moment has been a long time coming, and you have been there since the beginning. I know a lot of your time was sacrificed on my behalf. Thank you for being who you are, and I truly appreciate your friendship and support.

This journey would not be possible if it weren't for Gladice Houston, the senior patient care technician who hired me for my first job in dialysis in 1985. Gladice, I was just a twenty-one-year-old kid, recently discharged from the United States Army four months before you hired me. I worked several odd jobs before attending a trade/technical school for medical assistant training, four months before applying at the Austin Diagnostic Clinic, as recommended by the school's job placement department. You must have seen something in me that I didn't see in myself. I had never heard of kidney dialysis before applying at the Austin Diagnostic Clinic, and you gave me the opportunity—though I had no previous experience as a dialysis technician—to train there with you. I will never forget your warmth, compassion, and kindness during my interview, orientation, and employment. When my grandfather passed away during my dialysis technician orientation, you let me return to Washington, D.C. to attend my grandfather's funeral. In addition, you graciously let me return to continue my training. Then in November of that year, when my daughter was born, you treated me like one of your own children, giving me the time I needed to spend with my wife and newborn daughter. Gladice, if you had not given me the opportunity to train as a dialysis technician when I had many challenges going on in my life, I don't know where I would be right now. I am truly indebted to you. Thank you.

A big thank you and appreciation to Ann Cioffi, RN. Whether you know it or not, you were very instrumental in my obtaining my nursing degree. Your countless efforts in getting my classes and books reimbursed by the Fresenius Medical Care Nursing program, as well as making accommodations to my work schedule to attend nursing school, was nothing short of amazing. I can't thank you enough. Ann, you have been more to me than just my supervisor; you have extended genuine kindness, warmth, friendship, and compassion, all of which has meant the world to me. I also appreciate your sharing the keys to your cottage in Rehoboth Beach for the several getaways I was able to enjoy. I am so fortunate to have met you on this journey of mine. Thank you.

Tamika, my little sister, my ride-or-die and business partner—to God be the glory. Thank you for reaching out to me several years ago to join forces advocating for end-stage kidney disease prevention and awareness. This has been an amazing journey with you. Being your partner and friend is the best thing that could have happened to me. I truly enjoy being your partner and friend. There are no words to adequately express my gratitude, and I know the best is yet to come.

To the Urban Kidney Alliance management team: founding Urban Kidney Alliance, Inc. has been one of the most satisfying and rewarding experiences I have had in my life. To our board members, Dawn Edwards and Jared Brown, thank you for volunteering your time and energy to be a part of an amazing organization. Both of you have been a blessing to the organization and in my life.

To the wonderful hosts who broadcast from the Urban Health Outreach Media Network's Facebook

Acknowledgments

page, thank you for your unwavering dedication in making Urban Health Outreach Media what it has become. Through your shows, thousands of individuals are being educated and informed about all things kidney disease, including kidney transplantation, home dialysis, peritoneal dialysis, and end-stage kidney disease initiatives and policies. Each one of your shows has made a huge impact on our audience, and I pray we can continue working as a collaborative team. I humbly thank each and every one of you.

David Krissman: man, you have been a blessing in my life. I thank you for your friendship, encouragement, and hospitality. I am also grateful to you for showing me a different perspective on filmmaking and writing—your friendship is invaluable.

One person I truly appreciate and thank God for bringing into my life is Laura Gayle, RN, who reached out to me on a limb through social media and kindly offered her assistance to edit my manuscript before sending it to the publisher. Laura, of course you know that writing a book is not an easy endeavor, especially if someone has a lot going on in their life. I am forever indebted to you for your editorial help, keen insight, friendship, encouragement, and ongoing support in helping me bring this much needed book to life.

This book would not be possible without the dedicated team at WaltersPublishing.com. To everyone at Walter's Publishing, especially Pierre Walters—thank you for helping me navigate through the self-publishing process, especially since I'm a newcomer to the publishing world. A special thanks to Rachel Mountz and Steph Spector for your amazing work in producing my book.

To LTC Robert Cunningham (RIP retired USA), I wish I would've had the opportunity to meet you. Your letter addressed to me on July 18, 1964 has definitely shaped my life as a man and human being. It definitely set me on the path of making the world a better place than I found it. Thank you for taking the time during the Vietnam War to write to me.

I would be remiss not to give a special thanks to all the people who supported and worked with me throughout this journey: Erin Wheeler, Juan Wood, Donnell Debnam, Rhonda Rice, Joe McPhatter, Sade Cutler, Cassandra Floyd, Chef Brian Bordley, Chef Oliver Hale, Chef Jahfrey Juvon, Bruce Sparer, Gale Bell, Paulette Scotland, Nuyen Muhammad, Rob Browder, Binah Kane, the team at American Association of Kidney Patients, Diana Clynes, Richard Knight, Paul Conway, and Erin Khale—thank you.

Acknowledgments

Finally, to the countless patients affected by kidney failure that I have had the honor and pleasure of meeting and treating, I thank you for trusting me with your care. Caring for patients with kidney failure has been the most rewarding and satisfying part of my life. I truly and humbly thank you and enjoyed serving you.

Glossary

This glossary defines words that are often used when people talk or write about kidney failure and its treatments. It is designed for people whose kidneys have failed and for their families and friends. The words are listed in alphabetical order. Some words have many meanings; only those meanings that relate to kidney disease are included. A term will refer the reader to another definition only when the second definition gives additional information about the topic that is directly related to the first term. The following definitions were sourced from *Chronic Kidney Disease*, a manual compiled by the National Institute of Diabetes and Digestive and Kidney Disease.

A

access: In *dialysis*, the point on the body where a needle or *catheter* is inserted. (See also *arteriovenous fistula, graft,* and *vascular access.*)

acute renal (REE-nul) failure: Sudden and temporary loss of *kidney* function. (See also **chronic kidney disease**.)

allograft (AL-oh-graft): An organ or tissue *transplant* from one human to another.

anemia (uh-NEE-mee-uh): The condition of having too few red blood cells. Healthy red blood cells carry oxygen throughout the body. If the blood is low on red blood cells, the body does not get enough oxygen. People with anemia may be tired and pale and may feel their heartbeat change. Anemia is common in people with *chronic kidney disease* or those on *dialysis.* (See also *erythropoietin.*)

anuria (uh-NYOOR-ee-uh): A condition in which a person stops making *urine.*

arterial (ar-TEER-ee-ul) line: In hemodialysis (see *dialysis*), tubing that takes blood from the body to the *dialyzer.*

arteriovenous (ar-TEER-ee-oh-VEE-nus) (AV) fistula (FIST-yoo-lah): Surgical connection of an *artery* directly to a *vein,* usually in the forearm, created in patients who will need *hemodialysis* (see **dialysis**). The AV fistula causes the vein to grow thicker, allowing the repeated needle insertions required for hemodialysis.

artery (AR-ter-ee): A blood vessel that carries blood away from the heart to the body. (See also **vein**.)

artificial kidney: Another name for a *dialyzer*.

autoimmune (aw-toh-ih-MYOON) disease: A disease that occurs when the body's *immune system* mistakenly attacks the body itself.

B
biopsy (BY-op-see): A procedure in which a tiny piece of a body part, such as the *kidney* or *bladder*, is removed for examination under a microscope.

bladder: The balloon-shaped organ inside the pelvis that holds *urine*.

blood urea (yoo-REE-uh) nitrogen (NY-truh-jen) (BUN): A waste product in the blood that comes from the breakdown of food protein. The *kidneys* filter blood to remove *urea*. As kidney function decreases, the BUN level increases.

C
catheter (KATH-eh-ter): A tube inserted through the skin into a blood vessel or cavity to draw out body

fluid or infuse fluid. In peritoneal dialysis (see *dialysis*), a catheter is used to infuse *dialysis solution* into the abdominal cavity and drain it out again.

chronic kidney disease: Slow and progressive loss of *kidney* function over several years, often resulting in permanent *kidney failure.* People with permanent kidney failure need dialysis or transplantation (see *transplant*) to replace the work of the kidneys.

creatinine (kree-AT-ih-nin): A waste product from meat protein in the diet and from the muscles of the body. Creatinine is removed from blood by the *kidneys*; as kidney disease progresses, the level of creatinine in the blood increases.

creatinine clearance: A test that measures how efficiently the *kidneys* remove *creatinine* and other wastes from the blood. Low creatinine clearance indicates impaired kidney function.

cross-matching: Before a *transplant,* the donor's blood is tested with the recipient's blood to see whether they are compatible.

D
diabetes (dy-uh-BEE-teez) mellitus (MELL-ih-tus): A condition characterized by high blood glucose (sugar)

resulting from the body's inability to use glucose efficiently. Insulin normally helps the body's cells use glucose. In type 1 diabetes, the pancreas makes little or no insulin; in type 2 diabetes, the body is resistant to the effects of available insulin.

dialysis (dy-AL-ih-sis): The process of cleaning wastes from the blood artificially. This job is normally done by the **kidneys.** If the kidneys fail, the blood must be cleaned artificially with special equipment. The two major forms of dialysis are **hemodialysis** and **peritoneal dialysis.**

- **hemodialysis (HEE-moh-dy-AL-ih-sis):** The use of a machine to clean wastes from the blood after the **kidneys** have failed. The blood travels through tubes to a *dialyzer,* which removes wastes and extra fluid. The cleaned blood then flows through another set of tubes back into the body.

- **peritoneal (PEH-rih-tuh-NEE-ul) dialysis:** Cleaning the blood by using the lining of the abdominal cavity as a filter. A cleansing liquid, called *dialysis solution,* is drained from a bag into the abdomen. Fluids and wastes flow through the lining of the cavity and remain "trapped" in the dialysis solution. The solution is then drained from the abdomen, removing the extra fluids and eastes from the body. There are two main types of peritoneal dialysis.

I. **continuous ambulatory (AM-byoo-luh-OH-ree) peritoneal dialysis (CAPD):** The most common type of peritoneal dialysis. It needs no machine. With CAPD, the blood is always being cleaned. The *dialysis solution* passes from a plastic bag through the *catheter* and into the abdomen. The solution stays in the abdomen with the catheter sealed. After several hours, the person using CAPD drains the solution back into a disposable bag. Then the person refills the abdomen with fresh solution through the same catheter, to begin the cleaning process again.

II. **continuous cycling peritoneal dialysis (CCPD):** A form of peritoneal dialysis that uses a machine. This machine automatically fills and drains the *dialysis solution* from the abdomen. A typical CCPD schedule involves three to five *exchanges* during the night while the person sleeps. During the day, the person using CCPD performs one exchange with a *dwell time* that lasts the entire day.

dialysis solution: A cleansing liquid used in the two major forms of *dialysis-* hemodialysis and peritoneal dialysis. Dialysis solution contains dextrose (a sugar) and other chemicals similar to those in the body.

Dextrose draws wastes and extra fluid from the body into the dialysis solution.

dialyzer (DY-uh-LY-zur): A part of the hemodialysis machine. (See **dialysis**.) The dialyzer has two sections separated by a **membrane**. One section holds *dialysis solution*. The other holds the patient's blood.

donor: A person who offers blood, tissue, or an organ for transplantation. (See *transplant*.) In **kidney** transplantation, the donor may be someone who has just died or someone who is still alive, usually a relative.

dry weight: The ideal weight for a person after a hemodialysis (see *dialysis*) treatment. The weight at which a person's blood pressure is normal and no swelling exists because all excess fluid has been removed.

dwell time: In peritoneal dialysis (see *dialysis*), the amount of time a bag of *dialysis solution* remains in the patient's abdominal cavity during an *exchange*.

E
edema (eh-DEE-muh): Swelling caused by too much fluid in the body.

electrolytes (ee-LEK-troh-lites): Chemicals in the body fluids that result from the breakdown of salts, including *sodium, potassium,* magnesium, and chloride. The *kidneys* control the amount of electrolytes in the body. When the kidneys fail, electrolytes get out of balance, causing potentially serious health problems. *Dialysis* can correct this problem.

end-stage renal (REE-nul) disease (ESRD): Total and permanent *kidney failure.* When the *kidneys* fail, the body retains fluid and harmful wastes build up. A person with ESRD needs treatment to replace the work of the failed kidneys.

erythropoietin (eh-RITH-roh-POY-uh-tin): A *hormone* made by the *kidneys* to help form red blood cells. Lack of this hormone may lead to *anemia.*

ESRD: See **end-stage renal disease.**

exchange: In peritoneal dialysis (see *dialysis*), the draining of used *dialysis solution* from the abdomen, followed by refilling with a fresh bag of solution.

F
fistula (FIST-yoo-lah): See *arteriovenous fistula.*

G

glomeruli (gloh-MEHR-yoo-lie): Plural of *glomerulus.*

glomerulonephritis (gloh-MEHR-yoo-loh-nef-RY-tis): Inflammation of the *glomeruli.* Most often, it is caused by an *autoimmune disease,* but it can also result from infection.

glomerulosclerosis (gloh-MEHR-yoo-loh-skleh-ROH-sis): Scarring of the *glomeruli.* It may result from *diabetes mellitus* (diabetic glomerulosclerosis) or from deposits in parts of the glomeruli (focal segmental glomerulosclerosis). The most common signs of glomerulosclerosis are *proteinuria* and *kidney failure.*

glomerulus (gloh-MEHR-yoo-lus): A tiny set of looping blood vessels in the *nephron* where blood is filtered in the *kidney.*

graft: In hemodialysis (see *dialysis*), a *vascular access* surgically created using a synthetic tube to connect an *artery* to a *vein.* In transplantation (see *transplant*), a graft is the transplanted organ or tissue.

H

hematocrit (hee-MAT-uh-krit): A measure that tells what portion of a blood sample consists of red blood cells. Low hematocrit suggests *anemia* or massive blood loss.

hematuria (HEE-muh-TOO-ree-uh): A condition in which *urine* contains blood or red blood cells.

hemodialysis: See *dialysis.*

hormone: A natural chemical produced in one part of the body and released into the blood to trigger or regulate particular functions of the body. The *kidney* releases three hormones: *erythropoietin, renin,* and an active form of vitamin D that helps regulate calcium for bones.

hypertension (HY-per-TEN-shun): High blood pressure, which can be caused either by too much fluid in the blood vessels or by narrowing of the blood vessels.

I
immune (ih-MYOON) system: The body's system for protecting itself from viruses and bacteria or any "foreign" substances.

immunosuppressant (in-MYOON-oh-suh-PRESS-unt): A drug given to suppress the natural responses of the body's *immune system.* Immunosuppressants are given to ***transplant*** patients to prevent organ rejection and to patients with ***autoimmune diseases*** like lupus.

interstitial (IN-ter-STISH-ul) nephritis (nef-RY-tis) Inflammation of the ***kidney*** cells that are not part of the fluid-collecting units, a condition that can lead to ***acute renal failure*** or ***chronic kidney disease.***

intravenous (IN-truh-VEE-nus) pyelogram (PY-loh-gram): An X-ray of the ***urinary tract.*** A dye is injected to make the ***kidneys, ureters,*** and ***bladder*** visible on the X-ray and show any blockage in the urinary tract.

K

kidney: One of the two bean-shaped organs that filter wastes from the blood. The kidneys are located near the middle of the back. They create ***urine,*** which is delivered to the ***bladder*** through tubes called ***ureters.***

kidney failure: Loss of ***kidney*** function. (See also ***end-stage renal disease, acute renal failure,*** and ***chronic kidney disease.***)

Kt/V (kay-tee over vee): A measurement of ***dialysis*** dose. The measurement takes into account the efficiency of the ***dialyzer,*** the treatment time, and the total volume of ***urea*** in the body. (See also ***URR.***)

M

membrane: A thin sheet or layer of tissue that lines a cavity or separates two parts of the body. A membrane can act as a filter, allowing some particles to pass from one part of the body to another while keeping others where they are. The artificial membrane in a *dialyzer* filters waste products from the blood.

N

nephrectomy (nef-REK-tuh-mee): Surgical removal of a *kidney*.

nephrologist (nef-RAHL-oh-jist): A doctor who treats patients with *kidney* problems or *hypertension*.

nephron (NEF-rahn): A tiny part of the *kidneys*. Each kidney is made up of about 1 million nephrons, which are the working units of the kidneys, removing wastes and extra fluids from the blood.

nephrotic (nef-RAH-tik) syndrome: A collection of symptoms that indicate *kidney* damage. Symptoms include high levels of protein in the *urine,* lack of protein in the blood, and high blood cholesterol.

nuclear (NEW-klee-ur) scan: A test of the structure, blood flow, and function of the *kidneys*. The doctor injects a mildly radioactive solution into an arm *vein* and uses X-rays to monitor its progress through the kidneys.

P
peritoneal (PEH-rih-tuh-NEE-ul) cavity: The space inside the lower abdomen but outside the internal organs.

peritoneal dialysis: See *dialysis*.

peritoneum (PEH-rih-tuh-NEE-um): The *membrane* lining the *peritoneal cavity*.

peritonitis (PEH-rih-tuh-NY-tis): Inflammation of the *peritoneum*, a common complication of peritoneal dialysis (see *dialysis*).

potassium (puh-TASS-ee-um): A mineral found in the body and in many foods.

proteinuria (PRO-tee-NOOR-ee-uh): A condition in which the *urine* contains large amounts of protein, a sign that the *kidneys* are not functioning properly.

R
renal (REE-nul): Of the *kidneys*. A renal disease is a disease of the kidneys. Renal failure means the kidneys have stopped working properly.

renal osteodystrophy (AH-stee-oh-DIS-truh-fee): Weak bones caused by poorly working *kidneys*. Renal osteodystrophy is a common problem for people on *dialysis* who have high phosphate levels or insufficient vitamin D supplementation.

renin (REE-nin): A *hormone* made by the *kidneys* that helps regulate the volume of fluid in the body and blood pressure.

S
Sodium (SOH-dee-um): A mineral found in the body and in many foods.

T
thrill: A vibration or buzz that can be felt in an *arteriovenous fistula,* an indication that the fistula is healthy.

transplant: Replacement of a diseased organ with a healthy one. A *kidney* transplant may come from a living *donor,* usually a relative, or from someone who has just died.

U
urea (yoo-REE-uh): A waste product found in the blood and caused by the normal breakdown of protein in the liver. Urea is normally removed from the blood

by the **kidneys** and then excreted in the **urine.** Urea accumulates in the body of people with **renal** failure.

uremia (yoo-REE-meeare-uh): The illness associated with the buildup of **urea** in the blood because the **kidneys** are not working effectively. Symptoms include nausea, vomiting, loss of appetite, weakness, and mental confusion.

ureters (YOOR-uh-turs): Tubes that carry **urine** from the **kidneys** to the **bladder.**

urethra (yoo-REE-thrah): The tube that carries **urine** from the **bladder** to the outside of the body.

urinalysis (yoor-in-AL-ih-sis): A test of a **urine** sample that can reveal many problems of the urinary system and other body systems. The sample may be observed for color, cloudiness, and concentration; signs of drug use; chemical composition, including sugar; the presence of protein, blood cells, or germs; or other signs of disease.

urinary (YOOR-ih-NEHR-ee) tract: The system that takes wastes from the blood and carries them out of the body in the form of **urine.** The urinary tract includes the **kidneys, renal** pelvises, **ureters, bladder,** and **urethra.**

urinate (YOOR-ih-nate): To release *urine* from the *bladder* to the outside.

urine (YOOR-in): Liquid waste product filtered from the blood by the *kidneys,* stored in the *bladder,* and expelled from the body through the *urethra* by the act of voiding or urinating. (See also *urinate*.)

URR (urea reduction ratio): A blood test that compares the amount of *blood urea nitrogen* before and after *dialysis* to measure the effectiveness of the dialysis dose.

V

vascular (VASS-kyoo-lur) access: A general term to describe the area on the body where blood is drawn for circulation through a hemodialysis (*dialysis*) circuit. A vascular access may be an *arteriovenous fistula, a graft,* or a *catheter.*

vein (VANE): A blood vessel that carries blood toward the heart.

venous (VEE-nus) line: in hemodialysis (see *dialysis),* tubing that carries blood from the *dialyzer* back to the body.

Online Resources for Patients

AMERICAN ASSOCIATION OF KIDNEY PATIENTS

14440 Bruce B Downs Boulevard

Tampa, Florida, 33613

Phone: (800) 749-2257

Website: https://aakp.org

About: As the oldest and largest independent kidney patient organization in the United States, AAKP is dedicated to improving the lives and long-term outcome of kidney patients through education, advocacy, patient engagement and the fostering of patient communities.

TRANSPLANT JOURNEY

21 Locust Avenue, Suite 2D

New Canaan, CT 06840

Phone: 1-203-972-3334

Website: https://transplantjourney.org

Contact: Jen Benson, Founder/CEO

Email: jbenson@transplantjourney.org

About: Transplant Journey provides compassionate one-on-one support and non-medical guidance to transplant patients and their families. Their knowledge is based on personal experience that they acquired during their journeys to transplantation. They permanently work with each person to provide information and patient empowerment for their families with an A to Z guide through the transplant journey. Transplant Journey has mentors with experience in all organ transplant areas.

KIDNEY SOLUTIONS

Website: http://kidneysolutions.org

About: Kidney Solutions provides podcasts twice a week and shares them via link or on Kent's Kidney Stories every week. All episodes are catalogued on the site, and you can listen anytime. Kidney Solutions also provides a Kidney Support Group on Monday nights at 6:00 pm CDT via Zoom link. The group is for kidney transplant recipients and those seeking living donors. Donors are also invited. To join this group, you have to provide an email address, and then you will be invited. Their transplant support group meets every Thursday night at 6:00 PM CDT. Anyone who has had a transplant or donated an organ, or is a family member or caregiver, is welcomed.

DADVICE TV

Website: https://www.dadvicetv.com/

About: Founded in 2018 and counted among the largest patient run kidney resources online in the world, DadviceTV advocates for better kidney patient care and early intervention. Every week DadviceTV hosts interactive video broadcasts with experts on Facebook and its YouTube channel covering various aspects of kidney health. DadviceTV wants everyone's kidneys to stay healthy and is committed to the awareness, prevention, and early treatment of kidney disease.

TB7 WELLNESS COACH

Website: https://www.facebook.com/TB7H.A.M

Phone: (443) 402-6246

Contact: Minister Brian Bordley

Email: Tb7wellnessoutreachministry@gmail.com

About: A wellness coaching program that helps kidney patients live their best life possible.

KINDNESS FOR KIDNEYS INTERNATIONAL, INC.

Website: http://www.kindnessforkidneys.org/

Phone: (202) 599-7394

Contact: Sharron S. Rouse, Executive Director

Email: info@kindnessforkidneys.org

About: An online kidney disease support group for patients with kidney disease/failure.

FOR KIDNEYS SAKE, INC.

Website: https://www.4kidneyssake.org/

Phone: (833) 479-990

Contact: Dawn M. Lowery-Dawson, CEO

Email: info@4kidneyssake.org

About: A non-profit organization designed to provide recreational events/activities for kidney disease patients living on dialysis, who reside in NYC and Long Island. They also provide financial assistance for prescription drug costs.

Printed in Great Britain
by Amazon